Animal abuse and unlawful killing

Forensic veterinary pathology

For Elsevier:

Commissioning Editor: Rita Demetriou-Swanwick / Joyce Rodenhuis
Development Editor: Louisa Welch
Project Manager: Andrew Palfreyman
Designer: Charlotte Murray
Illustration Manager: Merlyn Harvey
Illustrator: Samantha Elmhurst

Animal abuse and unlawful killing
Forensic veterinary pathology

Ranald Munro BVMS, MSc, DVM, Dip Forensic Medicine, DipECVP, MRCVS

Professor of Forensic Veterinary Pathology
Royal Veterinary College, London, UK

Honorary Fellow
The University of Edinburgh Veterinary School, UK

Helen M. C. Munro BVMS, MRCVS

Honorary Fellow
The University of Edinburgh Veterinary School, UK

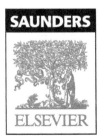

SAUNDERS

ELSEVIER

Edinburgh London New York Oxford Philadelphia St Louis Sydney Toronto 2008

SAUNDERS
ELSEVIER

© 2008, Elsevier Limited. All rights reserved.

First published 2008

ISBN: 978-0-7020-2878-6

British Library Cataloguing in Publication Data
A catalogue record for this book is available from the British Library

Library of Congress Cataloging in Publication Data
A catalog record for this book is available from the Library of Congress

ELSEVIER your source for books, journals and multimedia in the health sciences
www.elsevierhealth.com

Working together to grow libraries in developing countries

www.elsevier.com | www.bookaid.org | www.sabre.org

ELSEVIER   BOOK AID International   Sabre Foundation

Printed and bound in the United Kingdom
Transferred to Digital Print 2011

The publisher's policy is to use **paper manufactured from sustainable forests**

Contents

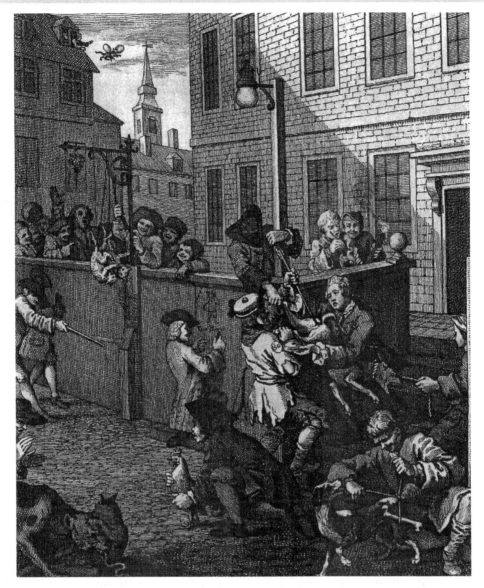

First Stage of Cruelty, 1751 (engraving) by Hogarth, William (1697–1764)

The Four Stages of Cruelty by Hogarth depict Nero's progression from cruelty to animals as a child through further cruelty to animals as an adult, leading on to murder and his final humiliation by public dissection.

Acknowledgements

The genesis of this book has been a long process that has benefited from the knowledge and common sense of many colleagues, not only in the UK but in many other countries around the world. To name them all would be a major task and would be fraught with the ever present danger of causing offence by an inadvertent omission. So we have chosen the global approach of thanking, most sincerely, all those who have assisted and supported us as we pursued the challenging task of developing a sound and 'science-based' approach to the emerging discipline of forensic veterinary pathology.

There are, of course, certain people who played a special part and deserve particular mention. We are most grateful to our veterinary colleagues in the Edinburgh University Veterinary School, The Royal Veterinary College, London (especially Professor Brownlie) and the Veterinary Laboratories Agency for their unstinting support for our work and for numerous discussions that we have had over the years. Our endeavours were enhanced by Mike Thrusfield's encyclopaedic knowledge of statistics, his good manners and sense of fun. Alisdair Wood's profound understanding of avian pathology and knowledge of firearms provided constant guidance (any mistakes are entirely ours!). Radiography has been crucial in the understanding of many cases and we have relied on the professionalism and attention to detail (often on extremely malodorous cadavers) by radiographers Rona Rae and Grace Paterson. Care and strict maintenance of 'the chain of evidence' combined with his good humour (and strength) made Craig Pennycook an essential part of the forensic post-mortem team at Edinburgh University Veterinary School. We also would like to thank Neil MacIntyre and his staff for cheerfully producing quality histopathology slides from many unpromising formalised samples. Craig Adam and Heather Darroch developed and printed the often gruesome images with skill and without complaint.

H.M. was funded by the Royal Society for the Prevention of Cruelty to Animals (RSPCA) to conduct the initial research into non-accidental injury, and this financial support was crucial to the success of the study. The Scottish Society for the Prevention of Cruelty to Animals also contributed substantially through access to records and cases. Special thanks are due to Phil Wilson, Jason Fletcher and Hamish Rogers of the RSPCA, and to Mike Flynn of the Scottish SPCA, for sharing their extensive knowledge of abuse of animals and providing guidance on the role that forensic pathology might play in the investigation of suspected abuse cases. The pathology of wildlife crime would have been virtually impossible without the enthusiasm and encouragement of Alan Stewart, Wildlife and Environment Co-ordinator in Tayside Police.

Introductions to pertinent German language papers were kindly facilitated by Dr Joachim Berchtold and Dr Alex Schock. Tremendous support for the dissemination of information on animal abuse, to veterinary undergraduates, was proffered by Intervet, and we are deeply indebted to Holly Cook, Sandra McLaughlin and Paula Boyden for their enthusiastic and thoughtful contributions. Elizabeth Ormerod generously shared her enlightened approach to cases of non-accidental injury.

Finally, we are most grateful to the following for permission to publish photographs: Scottish SPCA (Figs 5.1, 7.7, 7.9, 11.18 and 14.1), RSPCA (Figs 6.31 and 9.1) and Leonard 'Sam' Mansley (Fig. 6.4).

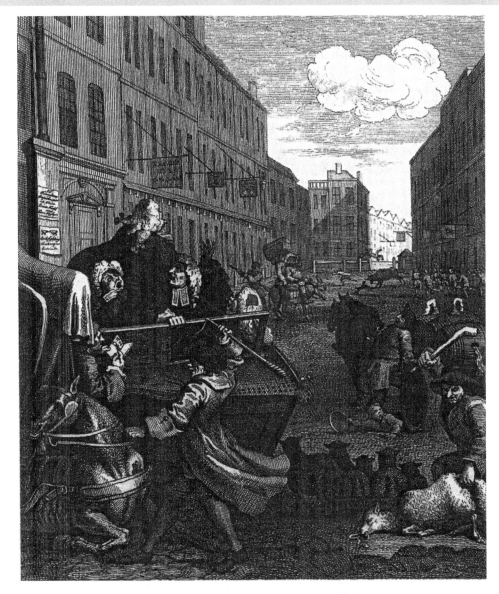

Second Stage of Cruelty, 1751 (engraving) by Hogarth, William (1697–1764)

Author's Note

Although I knew from a very early age that I wished to be a vet, where exactly that would lead me was never certain. However, the *raison d'être* was clear: to care for and to attempt to improve the lot of the animals. Specialisation in forensic pathology was not an early aspiration! Yet, through the opportunities that arose when living and working in East Africa, Hong Kong and the South Pacific, my interests in forensic veterinary pathology were kindled and early experiences gained.

The veterinary profession has an overriding responsibility for the animals under its care. The animals have no voice. They need advocates to speak up on their behalf to ensure that they are well treated. In this, forensic pathology plays a crucial role. When Cicero (106–43 BC) said *'Cum tacent, clamant'* [When they are silent, they cry out], he probably wasn't thinking in terms of forensic veterinary pathology, but the quotation is apposite. The investigation of animal cadavers provides insights into foregoing events that are difficult to gain by other means.

Abuse and unlawful killing of domestic and free-living animals is commonplace. Suffering in animals is often largely ignored despite many countries having laws to curb the worst excesses. Enforcement of these laws can be difficult or lackadaisical. At first sight this appears a depressing and hopeless picture, but the opposite is the case. Forensic veterinarians have a crucial role. Accurate investigation and balanced reports that present findings to the courts for decision-making support the application of the law and ensure justice. This is the way in which society advances because, in the words of Aristotle (384–322 BC), 'It is in justice that the ordering of society is centred'.

Ranald Munro
Edinburgh 2008

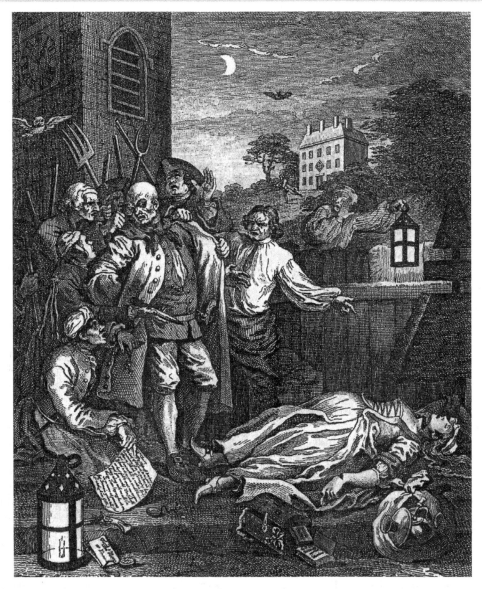

Cruelty in Perfection, from *The Four Stages of Cruelty*,
1751 (engraving) by Hogarth, William (1697–1764)

Author's Note

In the late 1960s, whilst still a very young veterinarian, I was asked to euthanase a kitten. This little animal had been left at the veterinary surgery by someone who had then departed the premises very rapidly.

When I examined the kitten it was apparent that something or someone had sliced off most of her tail, leaving only an open stump with clean incised edges. Unsurprisingly, she was somewhat defensive and distinctly unfriendly.

Some time later, a mother and daughter presented their large dog for examination. This patient had deep burns over her back and shoulders, and it was clear from the state of the wounds that they had happened several days earlier. I realised that the owners (who appeared to be mother and daughter) were 'uneasy' but, preoccupied with tending to the patient, I accepted the history that the dog had jumped up to the stove and knocked off a pan of hot liquid that had poured down over her. The owners apologised for not bringing in the dog earlier, saying that they had not realised how severe the burns were. Their uneasiness, I thought, could easily be explained by feelings of guilt about the delay. But something nagged at the back of my mind and only later did I realise the reason. Why, if this dog had jumped up to the stove, were the injuries over her back and shoulders? It would seem much more likely that the liquid would have poured down over her front paws and chest. A question formed in my mind. Had these burns genuinely been accidental? Or could it actually be possible that someone had scalded her deliberately? But I did not know if anything should, or even could, be done, and also doubted whether more senior colleagues would be helpful if asked for advice. The case of the kitten appeared straightforward: something or someone one had sliced off her tail. The dog, however, was very different.

Over the next few years I experienced more cases, some clearcut – such as a cat witnessed being thrown on to a bonfire – but also a few that raised yet again feelings of doubt and concern. Were the injuries really just accidents? And if they *were* caused deliberately, how could you differentiate them from *genuine* accidents? Clearly, if they were deliberate, an animal welfare problem existed, and my primary duty was to the animal.

More than 30 years later, and having specialised in a subject that had taken me away from clinical work – pathology – I read a paper by Phil Arkow in the *Journal of the American Veterinary Association*. His paper outlined increasing evidence – albeit anecdotal – that a link existed between violence to animals and violence to people (both adults and children), and that veterinarians were important because they actually saw and treated abused animals in their offices. Interested, I began to read more widely around the subject of violence and found myself including information on violence to children by caregivers. A paper written by James Stuart Hutton in 1983 was brought to my attention. The author, a senior social worker, suggested that evidence of animal abuse (of any type) might be a useful early diagnostic indicator of abuse to other members of the family. And my searches eventually led to a very famous paper in the *Journal of the American Medical Association*. Authored in 1962 by an American physician, Dr Henry Kempe and his colleagues, this paper described 'The battered-child syndrome', and documented the cases of hundreds of children who had been deliberately injured by their parents. The date of the paper showed that it had been written only a few years before I had seen the kitten with the wounded tail and the scalded dog.

Further exploration of child abuse literature told me that in the years that followed publication of the 'Battered child' the medical profession had developed guidelines to help to differentiate between *accidental* and *non-accidental* injuries in children. I thought of the kitten and the scalded dog, and of other animals that had raised concerns in my mind in the years afterwards. It was exactly then that realisation dawned on me – almost with a clang – that similar guidelines were needed for the veterinary profession, which was by now more than 30 years behind the medical profession. If the medical profession could do this for the welfare of children, so could the veterinary profession for the welfare of animals. In addition, and very importantly, if the abuse of an animal was to be used as a possible indicator of other family abuse then we needed to be able to *recognise* the abuse – in particular, deliberate abuse (non-accidental injury).

Thus it was that, with my colleague Michael Thrusfield (a veterinary epidemiologist who very deftly steered me, the veterinary pathologist, in the right direction with regard to numbers), I embarked on a large study of non-accidental injury in the dog and cat, as reported by the experiences of anonymous veterinarians in companion animal practice in the UK. Anonymity was considered essential because we wanted to encourage as many responses as possible on what was clearly a sensitive subject.

The study resulted in guidelines (described in Chapter 3) to help differentiate between non-accidental and accidental injuries in companion animals. These guidelines bear strong similarities to those established for children. On reflection, this is hardly surprising because there is a simple common factor: the person inflicting the injuries – the human perpetrator.

It is hoped that others will be encouraged to study non-accidental injury in veterinary patients. We are just at the beginning. There is far more work to be done.

Helen M C Munro
Edinburgh 2008

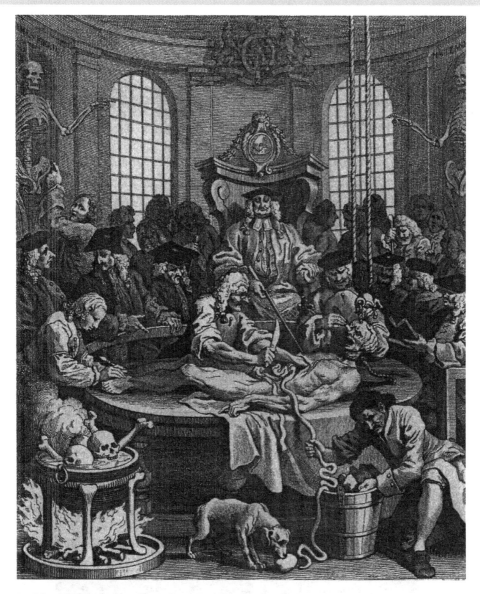

The Reward of Cruelty, from *The Four Stages of Cruelty*,
1751 (etching and engraving) by Hogarth, William (1697–1764)

Dedicated to Milly

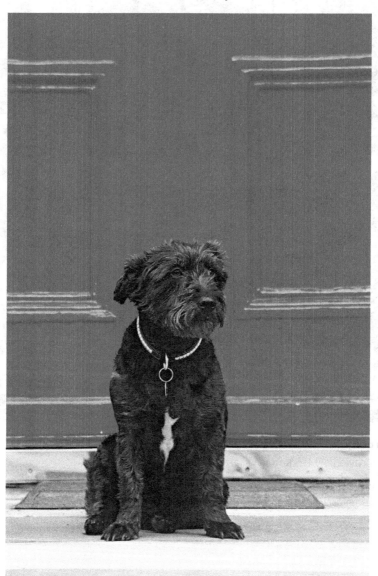

A survivor of abuse

1 | Introduction

'They [pathologists] form, of course, the
supreme court of diagnosis'

(Dr Theodore Dalrymple, 2001[1])

Forensic veterinary pathology is defined as the application of knowledge of veterinary pathology to the elucidation of evidence for the Courts. In other words, the purpose of conducting a forensic examination is: (a) to discover and record any injury, disease or abnormality, and (b) to interpret these findings in a manner that allows a Court of Law to understand the cause(s) and significance of any changes.

Forensic pathology is a highly skilled task, and veterinarians undertaking forensic post-mortem examinations must be able to demonstrate that they are competent in this field. As part of their studies at university or veterinary college, veterinary students learn the basics of post-mortem examination, but this is a meagre basis for claiming competence in a very difficult discipline. After graduation, few practising veterinarians take further qualifications in pathology. Consequently, although their clinical skills and experience develop with time, their knowledge of (and competence in) pathology is at best static. The end-result is that many veterinarians who undertake post-mortem examinations are at serious risk of presenting evidence that is incomplete, unconvincing or inaccurate. This is unwise in a professional sense. More importantly, the Courts may be misled.

The forensic pathologist is not required to 'prove' anything, but has the immensely responsible position of ensuring that the Court is presented with a comprehensive and as clear as possible picture of what has happened to the animal. Ideally, the forensic veterinarian should have a background in general diagnostic pathology. Without such experience of natural disease the task of guiding the Court in matters that might result in a criminal or civil conviction is made more difficult.

Microscopic examination (histopathology) of tissue samples is an important procedure in the diagnosis of disease. However, its use in forensic cases is generally limited. The veterinary aspects of the majority of forensic cases will be decided on gross lesions, rather than microscopic changes, and whether they match with other evidence in the case. There are particular circumstances where forensic histopathology can give convincing supportive evidence (see, for example, Chapter 9: Asphyxia and drowning). Nevertheless, in the current state of knowledge, care should be exercised about placing reliance on microscopic findings for assisting with, for example, the precise estimation of time since death and duration of injury.

This book is based on the combined and extensive experience of the authors but it is not comprehensive. Coverage is limited to the areas of forensic veterinary pathology in which we have been involved, and detailed comment on specialist spheres (e.g. equine work) that do not fall within our expertise is avoided. Nevertheless, much of the information in this book is applicable to the examination of a wide range of animals.

Guidance is provided on how to conduct a forensic examination, how to avoid some of the pitfalls, and how to assist the Courts in understanding the significance of some of the more common injuries and animal ailments. We have attempted to arrange the chapters so that the busy veterinarian or lawyer (or others) may find the key issues easily. Case examples with brief summaries of findings and interpretations are included, and we hope that this is helpful.

One of the major differences between veterinary and medical forensic pathology is the sheer number of species of animals and birds that the veterinarian might be asked to examine. To be knowledgeable about all of them is an impossible expectation. However, establishing contacts with specialists, who can provide advice on species identification, feeding habits, anatomy, diseases, etc., can partially redress this difficulty. Unfortunately, there are also many gaps in the current knowledge on forensic veterinary pathology. As the interest in forensic matters continues to build, these gaps will decrease but, in the meantime, the absence of detailed accounts of tissue reactions or lesions found in specific circumstances may be perplexing. The pathologist must, therefore, be constantly aware of the limitations and be prepared to advise that findings are inconclusive or are open to alternative interpretation. This can be disconcerting for the legal profession, which relies on veterinary guidance – but that is a legal problem not a veterinary one.

As in all specialities, terminology is important – and is particularly crucial when dealing with the Courts. In general, Courts are familiar with 'human' terminology and it is usually helpful if the veterinarian, when giving evidence, adheres to accepted medical terms. An example is the confusion that can arise when veterinarians use a word such as 'laceration' when, in fact, they are describing an 'incised wound'. Equally important is the avoidance, whenever possible, of technical terms. Latin or Greek names may be precise in a medical sense, but actually make no sense to the legal teams, judge or jury. When writing this book we have tried to limit the use of jargon so that it may be understandable to a wide audience. Similarly, the definitions provided in Chapter 2 (Fundamentals of animal abuse) are valuable in overcoming misunderstandings regarding classification and separation of the different types of abuse.

Insurance claims, over the cause of injury or the onset of disease in purchased animals, are usually civil matters and may depend on the balance of probabilities rather than 'beyond reasonable doubt'. But for the pathologist the task is the same: meticulous records, care and attention to detail, clear reporting and recognition that the veterinary report is produced to help the Court arrive at a just decision.

Reference

1. Dalrymple T. The odd psychology of pathologists. Sunday Telegraph 4 Feb 2001.

2 | Fundamentals of Animal Abuse

Classification of abuse

Confusion frequently surrounds the words 'animal abuse', because they are used to encompass a great variety of circumstances. In addition, other terms, such as 'animal cruelty', 'maltreatment' or 'ill treatment' are also widespread.

Veterinarians are aware (sometimes uneasily) that a further complication lies in the fact that the question of whether a situation or act involving an animal is judged 'abusive' also depends on the views that human society holds on *particular groups* of animals. For example, attitudes on what is accepted as tolerable regarding the husbandry and slaughter of farm livestock, the trapping and poisoning of animal 'vermin', and the use of laboratory animals in scientific research are quite different from what would be regarded as acceptable in the family pets. In other words, treatment that is commonly tolerated in one group of animals might well be considered 'abusive' in another.

However, in *companion animals*, confusion can easily and simply be avoided by applying the tried and tested typology developed successfully by the medical profession for *child abuse*. It can also be used in *appropriate* cases in all other animal groups.

Advantages of the typology

- It is simple.
- It allows a common language between veterinarians and other health professionals, such as paediatricians or child protection personnel.
- It reinforces consensus on *consistent terminology*, which is an important factor when carrying out research in this difficult field. Without the use of standard definitions, it is difficult to compare research conducted by different research teams.

The typology consists of four basic types of abuse: physical, sexual and emotional abuse, and neglect. More than one type may coexist.

Physical abuse

Synonyms:
non-accidental injury (NAI); battered pet syndrome

The perpetrator of physical abuse subjects the animal to a variety of actions that cause bodily injury. In some cases the fact that deliberate physical abuse has taken place is perfectly clear. A man witnessed beating his dog to death with a hammer would be such an instance. In others it is much less straightforward, and therefore can be much more difficult to recognise and diagnose. (See Chapter 3: Non-accidental injury.)

Figures from the Royal Society for the Prevention of Cruelty to Animals (RSPCA) in England and Wales for offences involving violence to animals show that violent acts are more often carried out by men than by women.

Sexual abuse

This means the use of an animal for sexual gratification. The term '*animal sexual abuse*' is preferable to the more familiar '*bestiality*' or '*zoophilia*', both of which focus primarily on the perpetrator, and thus fail to convey any sense of the physical harm that may occur to the animal. (See Chapter 14: Sexual abuse of animals.)

It is the very fact that the abuse involves the sexual organs or anus/rectum that distinguishes the abuse as sexual in nature. Physical injury to animals (or birds) of either sex may result and, depending on the actual type of sexual act carried out, and the size of the animal, can be very severe.

Emotional abuse

Although some might claim that animals have no emotions, and therefore cannot be emotionally abused, it is difficult to believe that veterinarians and animal behaviour specialists would agree. For example, regular threatening behaviour and verbal harassment of the animal (shouts, angry gestures), or a failure to provide psychological comfort, clearly constitute emotional abuse. However, neither author of this textbook makes any claim to expertise in this area, belonging as it does to the realm of specialists in animal behaviour. It is therefore not a subject of discussion here.

Neglect

This simply means a failure to provide the animal with the basic physical necessities of life: food, water and shelter. It also includes failure to seek veterinary attention for injury *and* for naturally occurring illness. Failure to provide veterinary attention in cases of natural illness is neglectful and falls within the definition of abuse.

Abandonment of an animal is a clear example of neglect, as is the all too common practice of allowing a collar to tighten and constrict the neck of a growing animal. Both men and women neglect animals, and it is common in all animal groups. (See Chapter 5: Neglect.)

'Intentional' and 'non-intentional' abuse

The law with regard to animals varies from country to country, and in some countries abuse is subdivided into *intentional* and *non-intentional*. This is not the case in Great Britain, because in both English and Scots law a lack of 'intention' to abuse is irrelevant under animal welfare legislation. In other words, it is not a defence for a person to claim that they did not intend to cause harm, or were unaware of the animal's needs. The factor taken into account by a Court of Law when judging a case is what a *reasonable person* would have done in the particular circumstances of that case.[1]

Animal abuse and the veterinary personality

Veterinarians tend in the main to be of the tender-hearted variety, caring deeply for the welfare of their animal patients but also frequently feeling compassion for the animals' owners. In addition, they mostly work independently, are accustomed to carry heavy responsibilities, and are recognised in their communities as persons of standing. All of these factors mean that it can be very easy for them to err by stepping outside their particular area of expertise (the veterinary one) when dealing with abused animals and their owners, and thus rationalise that particular circumstances mean that the perpetrators simply did not *intend* to be abusive. For example, they may consider that plain and simple ignorance of the needs of the animal has resulted in neglect. Or they may be aware that the owner has a particularly stressful home environment, and can therefore be excused a certain amount of violence towards a pet who has further stressed them by 'inappropriate elimination' in the home. In the first scenario, good advice may eliminate the problem, although this clearly depends on the level of neglect involved. In the violent scenario, it is unacceptable for the veterinarian to take it upon themselves to act as judge and jury when presented with any animal that has been injured deliberately.

Veterinarians need, therefore, to remember that their primary responsibility is to the animal. They can also be reassured that it is not their responsibility to *prove* abuse (of any type), because their responsibility is solely to provide relevant veterinary evidence. The final decision is not a veterinary one, but belongs to the Law Courts, where *all* the evidence and circumstances of the case are considered.

Medical knowledge of child abuse is helpful

It comes as a surprise to learn that the medical profession's acknowledgement of the very existence of deliberate injury of children by their parents or carers is relatively recent, coming only after a group of conscientious and courageous American physicians, led by Dr Henry Kempe, published the classic paper 'The battered-child syndrome' in 1962.[2] Exasperated by their profession's intransigence in acknowledging child physical abuse, Kempe and his colleagues gave their paper a deliberately emotive title, with the straightforward aim of attracting attention. The tactic was hugely successful, and in the USA an explosion in research on child abuse (of all types) followed. In the 45 years since this groundbreaking paper not only is the existence of child abuse widely accepted, but an enormous amount of knowledge on the subject has developed. Entire journals and textbooks are devoted to child abuse,[3–5] including a specialist textbook specifically on diagnostic imaging.[6] 'Diagnostic guidelines' to aid the recognition of child abuse in general – and physical abuse in particular – are now well established.

There is never any point in beginning from scratch and reinventing the wheel, and research has shown that the veterinary profession can make use of this medical knowledge because it provides an excellent base on how to approach the study of abuse (especially physical abuse) in four-legged patients.[7] Truly, there can be no more suitable subject for the modern concept of 'one medicine'.

The link between violence to animals and violence to people

Evidence, albeit sometimes decried as anecdotal, that there is a link between violence to animals and violence to people has been growing for some years.[8] In 1994 Arkow wrote that veterinarians have an important role to play, because they see and treat abused animals.[9] Further, he considered that not only do veterinarians have an ethical responsibility to the animal but also a wider social responsibility *'to take a leadership role in preventing abusive interrelations'*.[9]

Hutton, in 1983, suggested that evidence of abuse (of all types) in the family pet might be a useful piece of intelligence for early identification of abuse in other members of the family.[10] Gillham (1994) underlined the particular difficulty in predicting and preventing fatal child abuse.[11] Child protection personnel who become aware that family pets are being abused – and are prepared to include its existence in assessments – may find it a useful and rewarding piece of 'early intelligence'.

Nevertheless, to be able to use animal abuse as an indicator requires the ability to recognise and identify the abuse. This may seem simple in cases of abuse by neglect. A thin, malnourished dog, for example, may be visible outside the home or seen by visitors. But the situation with regard to recognition of *non-accidental injury* can be much more complex. Veterinarians in particular have invariably felt that they were in a difficult and uncomfortable situation when they suspected deliberate injury in a patient because, unlike the medical profession, the knowledge to help to differentiate the purely accidental injury from deliberate injury was simply not available.

However, research in recent years has helped to establish basic 'diagnostic pointers' for the recognition of NAI in dogs and cats, and these are discussed in detail in Chapter 3. These pointers – which may also be referred to as 'features' or 'indicators' – were developed from a study of the experiences of 1000 anonymous veterinarians in small animal practice in the UK.[12] A similar study, based on the UK model, was conducted in the Republic of Ireland[13] and produced comparable results.

References

1. Radford M. Cruelty: culpability and consequences. In: Animal welfare law in Britain: regulation and responsibility. Oxford: Oxford University Press; 2001:221–258.
2. Kempe CH, Silverrman FN, Steele BF et al. The battered-child syndrome. J Am Med Assoc 1962; 181:17–24.
3. Wolfe DA, editor-in-chief. Child Abuse & Neglect: The International Journal. Official publication of the International Society for Prevention of Child Abuse and Neglect. Oxford: Elsevier.
4. Meadow R, ed. ABC of child abuse, 3rd edn. London: BMJ Publishing Group; 1997.
5. Hobbs CJ, Hanks HGI, Wynne JM. Child abuse and neglect: a clinician's handbook, 2nd edn. London: Churchill Livingstone; 1999.
6. Kleinman PK. Diagnostic imaging of child abuse, 2nd edn. St Louis: Mosby; 1998.
7. Munro HMC, Thrusfield MV. 'Battered pets': non-accidental physical injuries found in dogs and cats. J Small Anim Pract 2001; 42:279–290.
8. Lockwood R, Ascione FR, eds. Cruelty to animals and interpersonal violence: readings in research and application. West Lafayette, IN: Purdue University Press; 1997.
9. Arkow P. Child abuse, animal abuse and the veterinarian. J Am Vet Med Assoc 1994; 204:1004–1007.
10. Hutton J. Animal abuse as a diagnostic approach in social work: a pilot study. In: Katcher AH, Beck AM, eds. New perspectives on our lives with companion animals. Philadelphia: University of Pennsylvania Press; 1983:444–447.
11. Gillham B. Fatal child abuse. In: The facts about child physical abuse. London: Cassell; 1994:41–67.
12. Munro HMC, Thrusfield MV. 'Battered pets': features that raise suspicion of non-accidental injury. J Small Anim Pract 2001; 42:218–226.
13. McGuiness K, Allen M, Jones BR. Non-accidental injury in companion animals in the Republic of Ireland. Ir Vet J 2005; 58:392–395.

3 | Non-Accidental Injury

Introduction

Synonyms:
physical abuse; NAI; 'battered pet syndrome'

Most injuries to animals are accidental and have no darker connotations. Nevertheless, many veterinarians are presented at some point during their working careers with patients whose case histories give rise to concern that their injuries are not purely the result of an accident. The Royal College of Veterinary Surgeons in the UK recognises this possibility and advises in the College's 'Guide to professional conduct' that '*When a veterinary surgeon is presented with an injured animal whose clinical signs cannot be attributed to the history provided by the client, s/he should include non-accidental injury in the differential diagnosis*'.[1] This chapter highlights the features that assist in the separation of accidental injuries from deliberate injuries.

Some cases of physical abuse are straightforward – for example, those perpetrators witnessed abusing animals in full public view. Others, however, are hidden, with the violence taking place behind closed doors at home. In the past it has often been assumed that owners who take their animals for veterinary treatment are unlikely to be abusive. This belief has been dispelled.[2]

It is these hidden cases that are sometimes referred to as 'non-accidental' injury cases, meaning simply that the injuries were deliberate and not the result of an accident. These are also the cases in which there can be real difficulty in making a diagnosis, not merely from an evidential point of view, but from a psychological one on the part of the veterinarian.

Difficulty of diagnosis

The diagnosis of physical abuse is not simple, and this is true for both the veterinary profession and the medical profession. The difficulties involved are particularly well described in the paragraphs that follow. The words were written for medical health professionals dealing with child abuse cases, but they also apply to veterinarians as they have the same doubts and fears as their medical colleagues.[3]

'*The diagnosis of physical abuse (non-accidental injury) is a difficult intellectual and emotional exercise. It is one of the most difficult subjects in clinical work, needing time, experience, and emotional energy. The biggest barrier to diagnosis is the existence of emotional blocks in the minds of professionals. These can be so powerful that they prevent the diagnosis even being considered in quite obvious cases.*

All those working with children [sic] should be warned that their overwhelming impulse on confronting their first case will be to want to cover it up.

The most important step in diagnosing non-accidental injury is to force yourself to think of it in the first place.'
Not only is the mindset of veterinarians and physicians similar, but also the similarities between the physical abuse of a pet and a small child are striking, the simple reason being that there is a common denominator in the shape of the human perpetrator. This means that the circumstances of the violence (perhaps someone arrives home inebriated), the actual acts involved (grab a puppy by the leg, or a child by the arm, and hurl it against the wall), the excuses offered (the kitten/child 'fell downstairs') and the resulting injuries (bruising, fractures, etc.) are, unsurprisingly, very similar.

Physical actions involved

The perpetrator subjects the animal to a variety of actions that cause bodily injury. These include kicking, punching, throwing (e.g. against walls, downstairs, out of windows), beating with an instrument, stabbing, burning, drowning and asphyxiation. Sometimes use is made of domestic equipment, such as microwave ovens, tumble dryers and washing machines, into which the animal is placed. The administration of drugs (e.g. narcotics or alcohols) and poisons (e.g. the slug bait, metaldehyde) also comes under the umbrella of physical abuse.

Species of animal

Although research on companion animal abuse has focused on the dog and cat, it should be remembered that other species of animals, including 'exotic' species, are kept as pets. All of these can be physically abused. It is also necessary to cultivate an awareness of the possibility of non-accidental injury in animals kept for *any* other purpose, for example farmed livestock.

Age, sex and breed of dogs and cats who have suffered a non-accidental injury

Dogs and cats aged less than 2 years are more at risk than older animals, and male dogs are more likely to be attacked than females.[4]

There is evidence that mixed-breed dogs and domestic short-haired cats are at increased risk, as are Staffordshire bull terriers.[4]

Disabled animals and disabled owners

It should never be assumed that a disabled animal will not be abused. For example, a deaf animal, appearing heedless of an owner's commands, may give rise to considerable frustration on the owner's part, with violent results. Similarly, it should never be assumed that support dogs, such as guide dogs, will not be abused.

Diagnostic features of non-accidental injury in pets

Particular features of a case raise concern that an animal has been physically abused. These features are also sometimes referred to as 'diagnostic pointers', 'diagnostic guidelines' or 'diagnostic indicators'.

It cannot be over-emphasised that no single feature is diagnostic; rather, it is a combination that raises suspicion, and this combination is variable.

Certain aspects in the history

For example:

- The history given for the animal is inconsistent with the injuries – the story given does not 'fit' with the injury. Usually the injuries are too severe to be explained by the history given by the person presenting the animal for treatment. An inconsistent history indicates that thorough examination and investigation are needed to confirm (or refute) any concern.
- The history is discrepant – more than one explanation for the injury is given, or the story varies from person to person.
- There has been a previous injury or death in another animal in the same household, or belonging to the same owner. Unexplained deaths or injuries are of particular concern.
- There is no history of a motor vehicle accident (MVA) or any other possible accident.
- The animal is housebound (many cats, for example, are kept indoors permanently).
- Family violence is known or suspected (Case study 3.1 & 3.2).

Repetitive injury

- This means that the animal is presented more than once with injuries, or different ages of injury are found on examination.

Case study 3.1

Male terrier-cross dog, less than 2 years old.

History:

The owner's ex-partner threw the dog against the wall. There was a history of violence towards the female owner.

Injury incurred by the dog:

Fracture of tibia.

Case study 3.2

Female domestic short-haired cat, over 2 years old.

History:

Both the cat and the female owner had been abused by the owner's partner.

Injuries incurred by the cat:

Severe facial bruising, bruising inside the mouth, and bilateral conjunctival bruising.

- The injury type may vary with each episode, but fractures feature prominently.
- Repetitive injury has a high index of suspicion (Case study 3.3 & 3.4).

Type of injury

- Multiple fractures in various bones, in different stages of healing.
- Some injuries may arouse suspicion because they are unusual, or do not 'fit' with the owner's explanation.

A particular person is implicated by the person presenting the animal

- Can be a partner or family member (including children).
- Can be self-admission by the owner.
- Someone else is blamed, e.g. a lodger, a neighbour or a stranger.
- The owner may say that he or she knows the injuries were deliberate but refuses to name anyone.

The behaviour of the owner arouses concern

For example:

- The owner may be reluctant to give a history for the injuries.

Case study 3.3

History:

Over a period of 3 months, three kittens aged 5–6 months were presented for veterinary examination. All three belonged to the same owner and all were housebound. In addition to being taken to the owner's own veterinarian, one kitten was twice taken to an emergency clinic and a second kitten once.

When first acquired by the owner, all three had been presented for routine check-ups and vaccinations.

A month after the routine examination, kitten 1 was presented dead on arrival at the surgery, having been reported to have 'stopped breathing' at home. Two weeks later, kitten 2 was 'found dead' at home. Kitten 3, meanwhile, was presented with a sudden onset of 'nervous signs' from which there was an eventual recovery. Five weeks later, a phone call to the surgery reported that kitten 3 was 'subdued', and 2 weeks later the kitten suffered a fractured spine, the cause of which was explained by 'a suitcase fell on her'. Kitten 3 was euthanased.

Post-mortem examination:

Post-mortem examination of all three kittens showed evidence of severe trauma. Kitten 1 had suffered a subdural haemorrhage, liver and kidney trauma, and a fracture/dislocation of the tail. There was also evidence of previous trauma in the shape of three healing rib fractures. The cause of death for kitten 2 was a subdural haemorrhage (see Fig. 6.15). Kitten 3's spinal injury was confirmed and the presence of 12 healing rib fractures plus extensive scarring on the top of her head confirmed at least one episode of previous trauma.

Salient features:

- The histories given to account for the injuries were inconsistent.
- Three kittens living in the same household suffered injuries. Two died from the same head injury.
- Repetitive injury had occurred: two kittens suffered at least two episodes of major injury.
- The kittens were housebound.

The outcome:

The female owner's male partner pled guilty to injuring the kittens.

- May be defensive or angry when questioned.
- May show a lack of concern for the animal.

The behaviour of the animal arouses concern

For example:

- The animal is frightened of the owner.
- Develops a fear of other people.

Case study 3.4

Mixed-breed dog, 1.5 years old.

Over a period of 4 months this dog suffered six limb fractures and three soft tissue injuries. On each occasion she was presented for veterinary examination. The man who owned her gave explanations that included statements she had 'fallen off a chair', 'been found on the floor lame', 'jumped off the furniture', 'run into a table' and 'another dog had run into her'.

Radiographic examination showed no pre-existing naturally occurring bone disease.

Salient features:

Inconsistent histories and repetitive injury.

- Shows a behaviour change (e.g. a friendly animal becomes aggressive).
- Is happier when separated from the owner (e.g. when hospitalised).

For comparison, pointers to non-accidental injury in children are summarised below. Note that, as with pets, it is a *variable combination* of these features that arouses suspicion.

- The history is inconsistent with the injury – usually, the injuries are too severe for the history supplied.
- The history is discrepant (i.e. changes in the telling, or from person to person).
- Repetitive injury.
- Unusual parental behaviour.
- Abnormal appearance or behaviour of the child.
- Certain patterns of injury (e.g. multiple fractures of different ages, 'fingertip' bruising, crescent-shaped [human] bite marks).
- The child may say something (although infants and very young children are unable to do so).

Fabricated or induced illness

Fabricated or induced illness (FII) is the current term for a particular and, it must be emphasised, *rare* type of abuse that is probably familiar to the reader by the older name of 'Munchausen syndrome by proxy'.

First diagnosed as a type of child abuse, it involves the falsification of illness in a child by a carer, the motivation being to gain attention and sympathy for the carer.[5] By convention, FII is usually allocated a separate chapter in paediatric textbooks.

In the veterinary context, the illness is fabricated or induced in an animal. A series of nine possible cases of FII were documented by Munro & Thrusfield,[5] who drew comparison with similar cases in children and emphasised the complex nature of this type of abuse, the diagnosis of which is '*acknowledged to be difficult and controversial*'.

There are different stages in this type of abuse, ranging from the giving of a fabricated history of illness in a normal patient, through a fabricated history with fabricated signs, to actual induced illness. By the third stage, a whole variety of physical signs may be induced, with the result that the clinician finds the case clinically puzzling and realises it is extremely difficult to draw a conclusion on the 'root cause' of illness. Recovery may occur if the patient is hospitalised and contact with the owner ceases.

Differential diagnosis

Clearly, it is essential to differentiate between injuries that have been caused deliberately and those that have occurred for other reasons. In this context, consideration should be given to naturally occurring disease and MVAs.

With regard to the former, veterinarians responding to a study of non-accidental injury in the dog and cat identified skeletal disorders and blood dyscrasias as factors for inclusion in the differential diagnosis.[4]

Skeletal disorders

Osteogenesis imperfecta ('brittle bone disease') is an uncommon hereditary disease that occurs in a variety of animal species[6] and should be included in the differential diagnosis of a patient presented with multiple fractures. Radiographic examination, ideally carried out by an experienced radiologist, is crucial, with normal bones on radiography eliminating the condition. Similarly, any suggestion of other bone disease, such as metabolic bone disease, will also be excluded. See Case study 3.5 and Figure 3.1.

Case study 3.5

A litter of young ferrets was found abandoned in a wood. Veterinary examination showed they were in extreme pain as a result of multiple fractures. Non-accidental injury was included in the differential diagnosis, but radiographic examination confirmed advanced nutritional bone disease (see Fig. 3.1).

The outcome:

The owner was formally warned about the neglect of the ferrets (which in this case combined lack of veterinary treatment and abandonment) and she was also given advice on the nutritional requirements of ferrets.

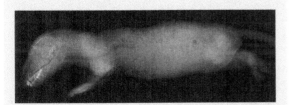

Fig. 3.1 – Malnourished young ferret showing severe loss of bone density.

Blood dyscrasias

When widespread bleeding or bruising is present, it is wise to perform laboratory blood tests to exclude any naturally occurring bleeding disorder.

Motor vehicle accident

These incidents are common, particularly in animals allowed to roam at will outside the home. They may therefore be a cause for concern for veterinarians when considering the differentiation of injuries caused by a MVA and those associated with suspected NAI.

It must be said that until additional data on the injuries associated with *known* cases of physical abuse are available there will be difficulty in differentiating abusive injuries from MVA injuries in some cases. Despite this caveat, however, there are several features to be considered.

First, it is important never to make an assumption of MVA. Many cats, for example, are housebound, making an MVA impossible. It should be routine to ask whether the animal is confined to the house and the response recorded in the notes.

Secondly, the body should be examined carefully for evidence of skin abrasions and dirt or oil in the hair coat, and their presence *or absence* recorded in the clinical or post-mortem notes. Any, or all, of these findings are often present when an animal has been hit by a vehicle. For example, in a study of 600 dogs involved in MVA, 79% had abrasions to their extremities and 35% had abrasions to their heads.[7]

Broken claws are often present after a MVA, and appear to be particularly common in cats (see Fig. 6.25). Again, their presence or absence should be recorded.

Fractures are common in both MVAs and NAI. Kolata & Johnson[7] recorded that, of 357 dogs involved in MVAs who had skeletal injuries, most of the injuries (302) occurred in the half of the body caudal to the last thoracic rib, with the pelvis being the most frequently injured structure (102). In contrast, a study of injuries associated with NAI found only one pelvic fracture in 147 cases of NAI where traumatic physical injury might have been confused with a MVA.[4]

Diaphragmatic rupture frequently occurs as a result of a MVA. However, this injury can also be a result of deliberate injury, and it is therefore wise in such a case not to make an *assumption* of MVA, particularly if other circumstances of the case suggest otherwise.[4]

Particular injuries associated with NAI

Modern textbooks on child abuse include weighty chapters on the types and patterns of injuries that raise concern of physical abuse, many studies having been carried out worldwide. An example is the child with multiple fractures of different ages, a feature of NAI[8,9] that also is applicable in animal physical abuse.[4] Another is the 'classic metaphyseal lesion' (CML), previously called a 'bucket-handle' or 'corner' fracture, as coined by Caffey in 1957.[10] A finding of CML is considered to be a strong indicator of abuse in an infant.[9] There have been no equivalent in-depth studies on particular types of injury associated with NAI in animals. Similar studies are needed, as much could be gained by their identification.

Key developmental milestones

Milestones in the development of kittens from birth onwards are well documented, and one milestone of key importance in cases of suspected NAI in kittens is the age of development of the 'air-righting reaction'. Development of the ability of a kitten to right itself while falling begins to develop at four weeks of age and develops smoothly over the next two weeks.[11] This means that by six to seven weeks of age kittens are able to turn over in mid-air and land on their feet: they do not land on the top of their heads. Consequently, explanations of 'falls' to explain severe head injuries, including skull fractures (which are commonly encountered in NAI cases in kittens), are highly unlikely to be accurate. This is especially true if the 'falls' are said to have occurred inside the home.

Developmental milestones may be relevant with regard to NAI in other species too, and could be a rewarding area for further research.

The approach to a case of suspected NAI

It is wise for all veterinary practices and veterinary organisations to be proactive. Ideally, it is preferable for an experienced clinician to be involved. Consideration should be given to the procedures to be followed and a policy should be prepared that is available for guidance for all staff. This particularly applies in larger veterinary practices, or hospitals, where an animal may be examined by more than one clinician.

It is extremely important to be objective, not jump to conclusions, and it is wise to remain calm, be polite, and avoid confrontation.

Note-taking must be thorough and comprehensive, and notes recorded clearly and accurately. All notes must be retained. Any (or all) explanations given to account for the injuries must be included in the notes, including explanations offered by different people. If no explanation is offered, this should also be recorded.

In the UK, when a veterinarian is presented with a case that raises concern of NAI, guidance to be followed is provided in the Annexes (annex 'c') of the Royal College of Veterinary Surgeons' 'Guide to professional conduct'.[1] Appropriate details for relevant authorities to contact are also included.

References

1. Royal College of Veterinary Surgeons. Animal abuse, child abuse and domestic violence. In: Guide to professional conduct, Part 3 – Annexe (c). London: RCVS; 2006. Online. Available: http://www.rcvs.org.uk 18 July 2007.

2. Munro HMC, Thrusfield MV. 'Battered pets': features that raise suspicion of non-accidental injury. J Small Anim Pract 2001; 42:218–226.

3. Speight N. Non-accidental injury. In: Meadow R, ed. ABC of child abuse, 3rd edn. London: BMJ Publishing Group, 1997:5–8.

4. Munro HMC, Thrusfield MV. 'Battered pets': non-accidental physical injuries found in dogs and cats. J Small Anim Pract 2001; 42:279–290.

5. Munro HMC, Thrusfield MV. 'Battered pets': Munchausen syndrome by proxy (factitious illness by proxy). J Small Anim Pract 2001; 42:385–389.

6. Campbell BG, Wootton JAM, Krook L et al. Clinical signs and diagnosis of osteogenesis imperfecta in three dogs. J Am Vet Med Assoc 1997; 211:183–187.

7. Kolata RJ, Johnson DE. Motor vehicle accidents in urban dogs: a study of 600 cases. J Am Vet Med Assoc 1975; 167:938–941.

8. Hobbs CJ, Hanks HGI, Wynne JM. Physical abuse. In: Child abuse and neglect: a clinician's handbook, 2nd edn. London: Churchill Livingstone; 1999:63–104.

9. Kleinman PK. Skeletal trauma: general considerations. In: Diagnostic imaging of child abuse, 2nd edn. St Louis: Mosby; 1998:8–25.

10. Caffey J. Some traumatic lesions in growing bones other than fractures and dislocations: clinical and radiological features. Br J Radiol 1957; 30:225–238.

11. Bateson P. Behavioural development in the cat. In: Turner DC, Bateson P, eds. The domestic cat: the biology of its behaviour, 2nd edn. Cambridge: Cambridge University Press; 2000:9–21 (citation of Martin P. Weaning and behavioural development in the cat. PhD thesis, University of Cambridge; 1982).

4 | Forensic Examination and Report Writing

The locus

In the context of forensic investigation, the 'locus' is the term used to describe the site or scene where the event occurred. Examination of the locus can help to place the incident in perspective and adds to interpretation of the post-mortem findings. However, unlike medical forensic pathologists, the veterinary pathologist is rarely invited to attend at the locus. More usually, the police or other investigators remove the cadaver from the crime scene and submit it for examination some time later. There may be little alternative in cases of wildlife crime where the incidents often occur in remote areas.

Nevertheless, it is advantageous if the veterinarian has the opportunity to examine the scene and gain at first hand an insight to the location and to the position in which the animal was discovered. Important issues, such as evidence of struggling, attempted escape or restraint, can be assessed at this time. When more than one animal has died or been killed, a site visit can be helpful in determining whether the deaths occurred at the same time or sequentially. Examination of the locus may also assist in placing the incident in a particular timeframe by observation of environmental clues associated with the body. The last two points are of relevance in, for example, investigations of suspected neglect of farm animals where cadavers are present in different pens or fields.

There are three basic types of loci:

1. *Incident, death and discovery at one site*, e.g. a collie dog is found drowned in a disused quarry with a rope and heavy weight around its neck.
2. *Incident at one site, death and discovery at another*, e.g. a hen harrier is fatally wounded by gunshot at one site but manages to fly to another location before dying and subsequently being discovered.
3. *Incident and death at one site, discovery at another*, e.g. a red deer stag is shot and killed by a poacher who then transports the body to a venison dealer's premises where the body is discovered following a tip-off.

General forensic procedure

The establishment of protocols for medicolegal investigations in veterinary medicine introduces a degree of standardisation that fosters objectivity and also encourages thoroughness. The use of a standardised protocol means that each case follows a routine, which, if adhered to, results in reliable documentation. The protocol should also include routines for radiography, photography, sample collection, labelling and storage of specimens. This may sound complicated but, once the system is set up and running, it becomes a routine that is easily followed.

No single set of protocols suits all circumstances, and each veterinarian, or group of veterinarians, should develop procedures that fit with their working practices. Best practice guidelines include:

- Maintenance of the chain of evidence by the provision of a receipt for the specimen when it is delivered to the laboratory or practice. (Evidence labels attached to the specimens should be signed at the time of receipt.)
- Recording of the specimen in the 'daybook' or computer system, and labelling of the specimen with a unique laboratory reference number.
- Creation of a document file, at the first opportunity, to record relevant details such as name of the person or organisation submitting the specimen (including any paperwork or labels accompanying but not attached to the cadaver), and contact details (e.g. telephone number and postal address).
- Availability of suitable, secure, storage facilities for the types of specimen being submitted. For example, small birds with delicate limb bones that are readily fractured post mortem should be stored separately from bigger, heavier specimens.
- Prevention of cross-contamination from one specimen to another by suitable leakproof storage bags/containers.
- Maintenance of a register of samples being placed in fridges or freezers dedicated to forensic work.
- Establishment of a routine for identifying, dating and signing radiographs.

Necropsy procedure

Preliminary considerations

The necropsy form

It is extremely easy, during a long and complicated necropsy, to forget to record details of an organ or sample. Consequently, the use of standard forms is recommended to prompt the pathologist to weigh and measure as required, to examine all systems and to take the necessary samples. Ideally, there should be a system of checking or corroboration that the procedures are being followed.

Receipt

When cadavers or specimens (including items such as dog collars or rings/jesses from birds) are received, a comprehensive history should be noted on the submission form. If, for reasons of confidentiality in sensitive cases, details of the circumstances have been withheld by the police, a note of this should be recorded. Similarly, comments such as 'received frozen' or 'in rigor mortis' should also be recorded, because questions may be raised about the state of the cadaver many months later.

A note should be kept as to the date and time of receipt, and what happened to the body immediately after receipt, i.e. was the body immediately necropsied, or placed in a cold store or in a freezer for examination later.

Public health factors

Some thought should be given to public health considerations and the possibility of disease, including exotic disease, before beginning the post-mortem examination. For example, imported psittacines transported in inadequate containers may well have died from hyperthermia or stress, but initial handling of these cadavers should take into account possible risks from diseases such as avian influenza. The use of a safety cabinet may be appropriate to safeguard the health of laboratory personnel.

Identification of particular species

The agency or person submitting a cadaver or specimen often identifies them in general terms (e.g. 'owl' rather than 'tawny owl' or 'short-eared owl') and it is advisable that the pathologist also uses the general term. This avoids any difficulties caused when different witnesses give different species names for the same specimen. It is also important to remember that in most cases, the veterinarian's expertise lies in the field of *pathology*, not taxonomy, so it is wise to avoid the possibility of making identifications that may cause one to look foolish later. However, if the veterinarian considers that the animal may have been wrongly identified then the submitting agency should be contacted and arrangements made for a formal identification by an appropriate expert. The expert should then attach an additional label bearing the correct species name.

Labels

Labels carrying the laboratory reference number of the cadaver are crucial to the maintenance of the chain of evidence and should be durable. Self-adhesive strips (12.7 mm wide) of industrial-quality, laboratory labelling tape, that is unaffected by freezing, with the laboratory reference number printed in black letters on a white background or white letters on a blue background, are easily read, conve-

nient and permanent. These strips can be placed around the leg above the carpus or hock joint, and can also be attached to other exhibits that form part of the evidence (e.g. a blood-stained baseball bat).

Some specimens may arrive with a paper or card evidence label that has been attached by the prosecuting authority or reporting agency. These labels, which are usually attached to the specimen by cord or string, can be protected from damage and contamination during the post-mortem examination by slipping them into self-sealing plastic bags and closing the bag mouth tightly around the cord/string. These evidence labels must be retained and are preferably left attached.

Removal of coverings

Any coverings around the cadaver (e.g. plastic bags, blankets, towels, papers or other materials) should be removed carefully one by one and listed. Identification marks or writing on the coverings should be recorded and any postage or transportation labels attached to the covering retained. Leakage of fluids should also be noted. The coverings may be malodorous and/or blood-stained, and it is not usually practical to retain them, but a careful search should be made for small objects enclosed within them, such as previously used submitting-agency identification tags (which have been removed), collars, leads or dogs' toys. These objects must be recorded and retained.

Body weight and length

After all coverings are removed, the body is weighed. The weighing machine used should be validated as accurate by regular calibration. The length of the body is then measured, a simple and convenient measurement being the length of the body from the back of the head to the base of the tail. (Weight and body size are particularly important in cases of neglect where the animal may have been deprived of nutrition.)

Photography of external surfaces

The external surface of the body is photographed on both right and left sides. Steps must be taken to ensure that the body carries identification (e.g. a pathology reference label) for each photograph.

Radiography

Whenever practicable, the cadavers of dogs, cats and other small companion animals and wildlife should be radiographed before necropsy.

External examination

A cursory examination will not suffice. The external surface of the entire body, including limbs, feet and ears, should be examined carefully, and any findings recorded. Maggots and beetles may be collected for forensic entomology. A general impression of the state of decomposition, bodily condition and evidence of burial (soil in hair coat) or immersion in water (body coat wet) should also be made. Detailed inspection allows description of particular colours (e.g. bruises) or marks (e.g. ligature marks on neck or feet), and the recording of sizes, shapes and positions of all lesions. Any skin disease is recorded.

Internal examination

The actual necropsy technique is a matter of choice for the individual pathologist, the important requirement being that the examination is thorough and consistent. Although the history may appear to point towards a particular cause of death (e.g. drowning, head trauma or poisoning) the post-mortem examination should include detailed examination of all body systems. This includes examination of the subcutaneous areas over the head, chest and body (for possible bruising), examination of the external and internal surfaces of the skull, and removal of the brain for examination. It goes without saying that all organs in body cavities are, after examination *in situ*, removed for detailed inspection. Leaving them in place will not do!

Changes related to natural disease should be recorded in addition to those that might indicate unnatural insult. Particular injuries (wounds, bruising, drowning, etc.) and specimen collection for specific forms of abuse (e.g. poisons, gunshot wounds) are covered in other chapters.

On completion of necropsy

Ideally, at the completion of the necropsy, all organs should be replaced inside the body, and the skin then sutured. Depending on the size of the body and the extent of the injuries, this can be a demanding task. Nevertheless, the pathologist has a duty to be respectful of the cadaver and of the sensitivities of the owner (who may wish to have the body returned); where possible, every effort should be made to ensure that the remains are presentable.

A record of where, when, and under what conditions the body was stored at the end of the post-mortem examination completes the post-mortem notes. The notes should then be signed by the pathologist and, if required, corroborated by the second pathologist. *There is no doubt that the better the notes taken at the time of the post-mortem examination, the better will be the report and any evidence given in Court months or years later.*

Interpretation of necropsy findings

There are two schools of thought over how much information the pathologist should have before undertaking a post-mortem examination:

- Should the pathologist study witness statements (if available), police reports and other documentation about the case before commencing the necropsy?

- Or should the examination be done before the pathologist gains any real knowledge of the background?

Undoubtedly there is merit in both of these approaches. In the first there is a danger that other people's observations and thoughts could skew the view of the veterinarian conducting the necropsy and that only those findings that support the preconceived ideas are observed. However, prior knowledge of the history of the case may well be very helpful, during the examination, in following a trail of events. Conversely, pathologists who commence the necropsy in virtual ignorance of the reported circumstances surrounding the case are unlikely to be biased and looking for particular features, but they may miss crucial facts.

On balance, it is better to gain as much knowledge as possible about the case before commencing the necropsy, but it is essential that an open mind is maintained and that meticulous recording of lesions, and normality, is standard practice. If all post-mortem examinations are tackled in this manner then the investigation will take account of possible causes of death (e.g. inhalation of smoke during a house fire), but will not fail to note bruising that requires a different explanation.

As mentioned above, interpretation of findings can be influenced by the alleged circumstances of the case, by interference with the evidence by others, by post-mortem change, and by lack of knowledge. The absence of specific knowledge about injuries and changes in animals and birds is an obstacle that must be recognised in forensic veterinary pathology. There is a multitude of as yet unanswered questions that can confound the inexperienced, the over-confident, and the over-cautious veterinarian. These uncertainties arise because of the huge variety of species that is presented to veterinarians and because detailed forensic examination of many of these species is a relatively new speciality. Problems range from lack of recorded knowledge, such as 'What circumstances lead to fracture of the hyoid in badgers?', to 'Do resolving bruises in dogs show the same changes at the same time as those in cattle?'. It is essential that the conclusions of the post-mortem report are balanced and honest. If there is a fundamental lack of knowledge about some aspect of the pathology then this should be stated clearly.

However, the Court relies on the veterinarian for guidance in the interpretation of the medical evidence. For the most part, the guidance sought by the Court is fairly straightforward. Examples are:

- Is it likely that a healthy cat would sustain a fractured spine by jumping on to the floor from a table?
- Did the fracture to the spine occur recently or some time ago?
- Would this cat have suffered pain and distress during the period between the incident and the time the cat was euthanased?

In this type of case, it is appropriate that the veterinarian should express an opinion. Not to do so would be an abrogation of responsibility. Particular care, however, needs to be taken not to stray out of one's area of competence or to express opinions on matters than are best explained by other experts. Pathologists need to avoid commenting on areas such as clinical treatments, statistics and animal behaviour unless qualified to do so as a result of recent training or experience.

Report writing

The post-mortem report serves three prime purposes:

1. It sets out, in non-technical language (see below), the normal and abnormal features found at time of necropsy.
2. It explains how these injuries or changes might have occurred.
3. It provides a balanced appraisal of the significance of the necropsy findings in relation to the case in question.

The report should have different sections (such as those below) that facilitate access to the information. A template for this type of document can readily be constructed and simplifies report writing.

Title page

The report reference number and/or the animal's name together with the name and address of the author of the report should be displayed prominently on the front cover.

Index

The various sections of the report are listed and numbered on the contents page:

1. Qualifications and experience
2. Instructions
3. Identity and administrative details
4. Comments and conclusions
5. Preliminary post-mortem findings
6. Post-mortem findings
   6.1 External findings
   6.2 Internal findings
   6.3 Samples retained
   6.4 Summary of findings
7. References.

1. Qualifications and experience
List academic qualifications and memberships of relevant specialist societies or associations. Give an outline of professional experience and current specialisation. Do not undersell yourself.[1]

2. Instructions
Set out who requested the post-mortem examination and what aspects were of particular relevance. For example:

'Sergeant William MacKenzie (No. 999) of Northern Constabulary requested that a post-mortem examination should be carried out with a view to:
   1. Recording any injuries present
   2. Establishing the cause of death
   3. Providing an opinion on whether the dog would have suffered pain and distress as a result of any injuries or disease before death.

Sergeant MacKenzie requested provision of a written report and inclusion of an album of photographs.'

3. Identity and administrative details
This section gives details of owner's name; name or identity of the animal; police or animal welfare incident number; species of animal; age of animal; sex of animal; colour or distinguishing marks; identity of person submitting the case; date, time and place of radiography; date, time and place of post-mortem examination, and persons present at the post-mortem examination.

4. Comments and conclusions
This section is often the part of the report that is of the greatest and most immediate interest to the person receiving the report. Consequently, rather than burying the conclusions at the end of the report, it is a convenience to place them at the front. Having read the conclusions and the comments, the reader can then pass to the detail of the post-mortem findings in the following sections.

A report that comes to no conclusion, or is greatly fudged with caveats, does not aid the Court, or other body assessing the case, in coming to an informed judgement. The veterinarian's job is to help and guide this process. Dodging the issues is a disservice. There are times when the veterinary evidence is inconclusive, but that should be stated clearly in the report. If the cause of death cannot be determined despite thorough investigation, the report should set this out unambiguously: 'The cause of death could not be ascertained'. If the case revolves around pain and distress, and the dog had a fractured leg, the report should be straightforward and state that the dog suffered at the time of the injury and during any subsequent period when veterinary treatment was lacking.

Body weight is an essential element of many reports and, if relevant to the formation of veterinary opinion, appropriate reference ranges for the type of animal or bird should be included in the report. Authentication is needed when statements on the duration of neglect are made. It is not uncommon to encounter general unsupported comments in reports, such as 'She must have been starved for weeks', yet the report's author does not have access to published peer-reviewed references that give objective guidance on how long it might take for this particular animal to lose weight, nor does the author know how much food was being fed. The fact that the animal was underweight and malnourished and had not been taken to the veterinary clinic for examination may be undermined by well meaning but unsupported opinion.

Opinion should always be soundly based and, if appropriate, supported by relevant reference to published literature. It is a matter of judgement which references are included, but the case must be balanced and fair.

5. Preliminary post-mortem findings

A short account is given of the date and time of receipt of the cadaver, where it was received, and details such as 'received frozen', 'placed in chill at 4°C' or 'allowed to thaw in an ante-room off the post-mortem room for 24 hours'. Details of the packaging, seals or identity tags are recorded here.

6. Post-mortem findings

6.1 External findings & 6.2 Internal findings

Recording external and internal post-mortem findings in separate subsections lends clarity to the report by ensuring there is no doubt whether particular lesions were visible on the surface of the body or located internally.

It is also extremely helpful if the paragraphs are numbered, as this greatly facilitates reference to particular findings. It should be made clear which organs have been examined; this can be achieved by simple notes such as '6.2.8 Thyroids: no significant findings'. If some organ or tissue that would normally be examined was absent, or was overlooked, this should be recorded, for example: '6.2.12 Left kidney: not present'.

6.3 Samples retained

Where tissue specimens are preserved or bullet fragments etc. are taken for further examination, these samples are listed in this section and details provided on what tests (if any) were performed and where these tests were conducted. For example, if anticoagulant rodenticide poisoning was suspected in a bird of prey, it might be noted in section 6.3 that gullet and stomach contents, liver and kidney samples (each in separate containers) were delivered to the toxicology department of a named institute for analysis. This section also records how the body was wrapped, sealed and stored on completion of the post-mortem examination.

6.4 Summary of findings

The main findings of the examination, without comment on their significance, are listed.

7. References

Selected references cited in the comments section should be listed at the end of the report, e.g. Harkin KR. Gastric ulcer. In: Cote E, ed. Clinical veterinary advisor: dogs and cats. Philadelphia: Mosby Elsevier; 2007:431–433.
NB: The report is not complete until signed and dated.

Style of writing

Your report is for the benefit of the Courts and should be written with this in mind.

A minimum font size of 12 point is recommended, and the report may be double spaced if wished.

Many reports contain veterinary medical terms and jargon. Although it is convenient for the veterinarian to use specific anatomical and pathological terms, it is entirely unhelpful for the lawyers, judges and other non-veterinarians who are required to read these reports. Descriptions such as 'comminuted' or 'horizontal ramus' detract from the usefulness of the report. Consequently (although it may seem strange, awkward, or even simplistic at first), lay terms should be used wherever possible. In place of 'comminuted' it might be better to write 'broken into small pieces'. Similarly, 'horizontal ramus of the mandible' is more easily understood as 'the horizontal part of the lower jaw bone that extends from the point of the chin to the angle of the jaw'. Words that are used frequently in human forensic cases may be appropriate (e.g. 'wrist' rather than carpus, and 'knee' rather than stifle). This makes the thrust of the report considerably more accessible to people who may be familiar with human cases but are uncertain about animals. The accuracy of lay terms can be ensured by adding the anatomical name in brackets after the lay term, e.g. 'The long narrow bones in the hind foot (metatarsal bones)'.

Care at the time of composing the report will be rewarded by avoidance of unnecessary discussion on ambiguous terms and the meaning that these words or phrases may have to the lay person. For example, 'starvation' is best avoided as, to many people, it implies that *no* food was available, whereas the animal's very poor bodily condition might have been a result of *inadequate* food rather than a total lack of rations. In such a case, 'malnutrition' or 'under-nutrition' properly describes the state of affairs.

The clarity of reports can be improved by the use of simple sentences that exclude doubt about specific issues. Examples are:

- 'Natural disease played no part in the death of this animal.'
- 'There is no evidence to suggest that this animal was rendered insensible.'
- 'The severity of the brain injury suggests that this animal would have been rendered insensible instantly.'

However, care must be taken to ensure that the report is balanced, gives an accurate picture of the known facts, and that negative issues are not omitted merely because they might detract from your opinion.

Part of the care in writing the report should also include accurate spelling, correct punctuation and good sentence construction. In the descriptive part of the report it is acceptable to record features of the pathology in note form, but in the section covering 'Comments and conclusions' the veterinary expert is expected to write simply and well.

Reference

1. Royal College of Paediatrics and Child Health. Practical points for report writing. In: Child protection companion, Appendix 16. London: RCPCH; 2006:A53.

5 | Neglect

Introduction

A neglected animal has been deprived of one or more of the basic necessities of life: food, water, shelter, veterinary treatment. Lack of veterinary treatment can apply to both injuries and naturally occurring disease.

Deprivation of emotional comfort is also neglectful, but is a matter for clinicians and specialists in animal behaviour and so falls outside the remit of this text.

Malnutrition

General

Malnutrition is poor nutrition that has arisen as a consequence of insufficient or poorly balanced food, or because of faulty digestion or utilisation of food.[1] Owners and keepers of animals have a responsibility to investigate the causation of any suspected malnutrition problem in animals under their care. Not to do so is neglectful.

Recognition of severe malnutrition is relatively straightforward and veterinary involvement is usually restricted to those cases involving gross neglect (Figs 5.1 & 5.2). Body condition scoring methods are available for different species of domestic animals and are subdivided for different classes of farm animal, e.g. dairy cows and beef suckler cows and heifers. These guides can be invaluable to clinicians as the veterinarian must have a thorough understanding of the variation in body condition that is the 'accepted norm' at different times of the year in the various livestock husbandry systems. Similarly, birds of prey that are used for hunting may have 'flying weights' that are significantly less than the ideal weight for a resting bird.

In *live* animals, body scoring provides a clear indication of the adequacy of recent nutrition. However, because these methods are designed to assess animals in the standing position, they are less applicable to cadavers. Additionally, alterations related to post-mortem degeneration may influence the body score. Nevertheless, before beginning dissection on whole fresh cadavers it is useful to palpate the body (in a similar manner to body scoring the live animal), in order to make a general assessment of body condition ranging from 'excellent' through 'adequate' to 'emaciated'. Whenever possible, the weight of the animal should be compared with breed standards.

Malnutrition, infection and the immune system

The interaction between malnutrition, frequent infection and impaired immune function has been the subject of much interest over many years. In human medicine the cyclical nature of this interrelationship, where each element has an effect on the other two, has been accepted for nearly 40 years following publication of the monograph by Scrimshaw et al.[2] Keusch[3] provided clarity, in 1990, regarding the manner in which these three factors can result in the downward spiral of bodily condition. These findings are equally valid for domestic animals.

In the past it was assumed that malnutrition was the primary cause that resulted in impaired immune function and subsequent frequent or persistent infections. There is persuasive experimental evidence that this sequence of events can occur.[4] However, infection (in the form of parasites or microbial infections) may be the initiating cause of the downward spiral in animals being fed a marginal diet. During infections the patient may have a reduced food intake, compounded by increased energy consumption, catabolism of muscle proteins, loss of nitrogen stores, and depletion of glycogen and fat stores. The animal moves from a state of marginal diet into protein-energy malnutrition. Without an improvement in diet, cell-mediated immunity is impaired and infections persist or recur before the immune damage can be repaired. Thus, the body condition of the animal continues to decline. Interventions to prevent the decline are dependent on improving various aspects of the husbandry to lift the animal from its marginal diet and reduce the disease challenge.

Post-mortem findings in malnutrition

Skin

There is loss of subcutaneous fat, and the skin may become wrinkled through dehydration. Protein deficiency leads to a dull, dry and brittle coat. Particular mineral or vitamin deficiencies may give rise to specific histopathological changes, e.g. parakeratosis in zinc-deficient pigs.

Muscle

Atrophy of muscle masses begins in monogastrics after 24 hours of starvation. In calves and lambs this change takes slightly longer, whilst its onset in adult ruminants is delayed for about 3 days. The back and thigh muscles are first

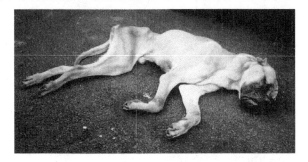

Fig. 5.1 – Bull mastiff. Neglected and starved to the point of death over a 5-month period. (By kind permission of the Scottish Society for the Prevention of Cruelty to Animals.)

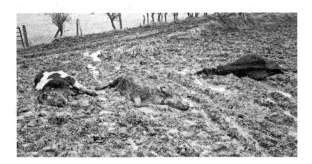

Fig. 5.2 – More than 20 dead cattle were discovered during the initial visit to a farm following a complaint by a member of the public. The remaining animals were uniformly malnourished.

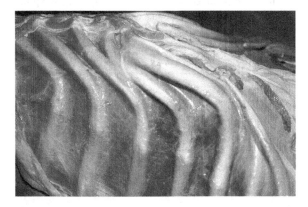

Fig. 5.3 – Bull mastiff (see Fig 5.1). Profound loss of muscle. The deformity of the rib cage allowed tracing of the breeder and the dog's owner.

affected but the process extends to all muscle groups (Fig. 5.3). Depletion of glycogen deposits in the muscle cells of emaciated animals interferes with the normal process of rigor mortis. Consequently these bodies do not 'set'.

Fat

The fat deposits in the omentum and mesentery are first to be depleted. Fat is then mobilised from other sites such as the perirenal area (the major deposit in adult ruminants), from under the skin, around the heart, and within the bone marrow. Fat is also lost from the connective tissue in muscle, resulting in a flabby appearance. 'Serous atrophy' is the term used to describe the gelatinous masses containing flecks of degenerating fat found in the perirenal and coronary areas of emaciated animals. These jelly-like deposits are formed as the fat droplets are removed and replaced by proteinaceous fluid accompanied by a general increase in interstitial fluid related to hypoproteinaemia. Histopathological examination may show droplets of fat in the loops of Henle in the kidney (experience is required when interpreting changes in cats) and in myocytes.

Chemical estimation of the percentage of fat in bone marrow has been suggested as a measure of the degree of depletion of fat reserves. Inevitably there are species, breed and sampling site variations related to this technique. In the authors' view this is an unnecessary test that merely adds complication to the practical assessment of the general state of debility. If chronic debilitating disease is absent yet the animal is thin, devoid of normal fat reserves and shows atrophy of muscle, then it is malnourished.

Stomach and intestines

In the normal, healthy ruminant, the rumen accounts for approximately 25% of live weight. The rumen of a markedly underweight animal may exceed this figure because of the loss of bodily condition and the consumption of quantities of poor-quality feed. The ruminal contents of normal sheep tend to be relatively dry compared with those of cattle, and the observation of moderate quantities of fluid in the ovine rumen is an indication of starvation and *not* that the sheep had been drinking water. The presence of food in the rumen is frequently advanced as evidence that the animals were being fed adequately. This may not be the case, because many severely malnourished animals have quantities of fibrous material in the rumen. Consequently, retention and analysis of rumen contents may be helpful in determining the nutritional value of the food available to the animal.

The observation of moderate quantities of wet, semi-solid digesta within the upper parts of the intestines of undernourished ruminants is sometimes presented as evidence of recent, adequate feeding. However, this could be misleading because the intestinal contents are the product of slow and progressive digestion of fibrous material in the rumen and eventual passage of this partially digested food to the remainder of the digestive tract some time after ingestion. As a result, starved ruminants commonly have quantities of wet or bulky intestinal contents.

Similarly, the copious sacculated large intestines of rabbits may contain considerable quantities of wet or fluid contents, even when the skin and the muscle mass of the body show signs of malnourishment and dehydration.

Dogs and cats do not store food in their stomachs for extended periods. In most cases, food passes to the intestines within hours of ingestion. Consequently, in contrast to ruminants, the stomach and small intestines of dogs and cats after several days of starvation may be virtually empty, or may contain only quantities of mucus. Gastric ulceration (Fig. 5.4), caused by reduced blood flow to the lining of the stomach, in malnourished dogs may lead to perforation of the stomach wall. Hungry animals may ingest a variety of indigestible materials (plastic bags, rubber, cloth, wood) and the stomach can become distended with this type of non-food material (Fig. 5.5). Dry or sticky faecal material may be present in the large intestine.

A notable feature of dogs and cats that have starved to death is that the gastrointestinal tract is often considerably less malodorous than that of adequately nourished and hydrated specimens.

Other organs

All organs atrophy as emaciation progresses, with the changes being most obvious in the liver, spleen, pancreas, thymus and salivary glands. Microscopically, the liver cells may show atrophy. The lymph nodes of young animals may, however, be enlarged and oedematous, and bone marrow may be red, watery and poor in fat. Radiography can be used to highlight growth arrest lines in the long bones of young animals.

Natural disease and malnutrition

Post-mortem examination of very thin animals may uncover natural disease or physiological states that could account, at least partially, for the poor bodily condition, e.g. advanced neoplasia (Fig. 5.6), Johne's disease, heavy parasitism, lactation. The duty of the veterinarian is to make an assessment of the contribution that these processes played in the reduction of body condition and to note whether appropriate veterinary treatment had been sought for the progressive loss of weight. These matters are not always clearcut (Case study 5.1).

Equally important must be the recognition that not all diseases or infections result in poor condition. For example, post-mortem examination of malnourished farm animals will frequently show evidence of limited areas of pneumonia and small numbers of liver flukes or lungworms. Such findings should be recorded and included in the final report, but if it is considered that they lack

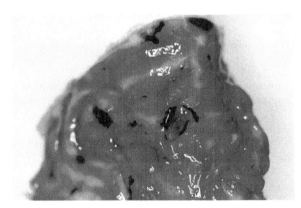

Fig. 5.4 – Gastric erosion and ulceration in a severely malnourished and hypothermic greyhound/lurcher puppy.

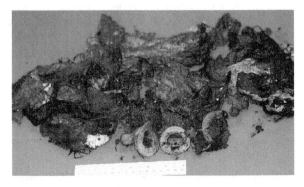

Fig. 5.5 – This severely malnourished 18-month-old Rotweiler dog died following perforation of a gastric ulcer. The stomach was filled with a mass of indigestible material including rubber and plastic.

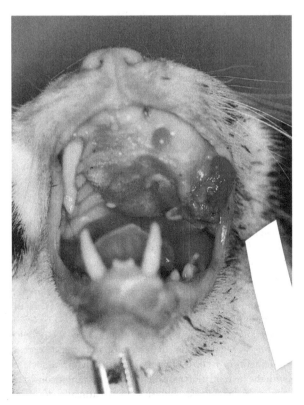

Fig. 5.6 – Emaciated adult cat showing advanced neoplasia in the roof of the mouth and protruding on the left side. No veterinary attention had been sought.

Clinical history:

'Peggy' was an adult Staffordshire bull terrier type. She died in late January. It was reported that she had puppies 'sometime before Christmas', but these had been found homes before the New Year. She had been fed at around 18.00 hours and was discovered dead the following morning.

Post-mortem examination:

Peggy was very thin but her weight was 13.5 kg, which falls within the breed standard (11–15.4 kg) for British Staffordshire bull terrier bitches. She had no omental or subcutaneous fat, contained no intestinal parasites, and showed no evidence of systemic infections, degenerative disease or neoplasia. Her nipples were prominent but the mammary tissue was inactive. The cause of death was 180° torsion of the stomach. The stomach contained 1.8 kg of proprietary dog food.

The issues:

Peggy was considerably underweight for her size of frame and her loss of weight would have taken some time to develop. She was clearly undernourished but the dilemma for the forensic veterinary practitioner lies in deciding what part her previous gestation and lactation played in her loss of condition. Should the owners have noticed her declining weight and should she have received veterinary attention? Death was related to feeding an abnormally large meal to a thin, possibly very hungry, dog. Was this a manifestation of ongoing neglectful behaviour or, perhaps, an inappropriate action by an ill informed owner who was responding to adverse criticism on the dog's body condition?

relevance to the decline in body condition this should be clearly stated.

Neglected injuries: general aspects

Accidents and misadventure account for an enormous range of injuries encountered in veterinary practice. Most are treated adequately, but some are not. A small proportion of the latter cases may be referred for forensic veterinary examination. Although species and breed differences can complicate the picture, there are features that are common to most of these investigations.

Details of when and how the injury occurred, and what actions were taken immediately, and later, can be crucial. Statements or records of interviews with people associated with the investigation may highlight important inconsistencies regarding times, clinical signs, treatments, locations and husbandry practices.

Case studies 5.2–5.5 (Figs 5.7–5.12) provide examples of different injuries and interpretations of findings.

Farm animal lameness

General

Lameness in farm animals is extremely common and 'is undoubtedly a major welfare problem'.[5] However, it is considered by many livestock keepers to be 'unfortunate' but that there is little or nothing that can be done about it. This common acceptance of farm animal lameness draws a distinction between companion animals and farm livestock with regard to what is considered as a welfare problem. Where treatable, but untreated, injury or disease in a family pet might lead to prosecution, many instances of equal severity in cattle, sheep and goats pass unremarked.

In addition to the clear animal welfare factor, veterinarians have responsibilities to society, because the public would not wish to buy products originating from farm animals raised in welfare-unfriendly conditions. It is therefore incumbent upon the profession to undertake thorough and objective investigation of cases of farm animal lameness. To do this, the veterinarian needs a sound understanding of the relevant anatomy and physiology and of the types of disease or injury that are encountered.[6,7]

Post-mortem examination of lameness in farm animals

Lameness in farm animals is a multifactorial problem in terms of both causation and pathology. Forensic examination can be invaluable in providing objective evidence on the nature and chronicity of lesions.

The forensic aspects of lameness generally fall into one or other of the following categories:

- Lack of veterinary treatment
- Claims (financial or welfare associated) related to cases of acute lameness, e.g. did the fracture of the leg occur during transport, or shortly after the animal arrived at market?

Irrespective of the underlying reasons for the investigation, the actual examination of the animal or specimen follows the same procedure. The veterinarian is required to determine:

- The changes present
- The pathogenesis of the lesions
- The time that has elapsed since the initial insult
- Whether there is evidence of veterinary treatment
- Whether the animal would have suffered unnecessarily during the progression of the disease or injury.

Although the investigation may involve the whole animal, it is equally probable that only the legs or feet will be submitted for examination. At the time of submission, each leg or foot should be labelled with the animal's ear-tag number

Case study 5.2: Neglect of post-calving injuries

Clinical history:

During a routine welfare visit by State Veterinary Officers, a filthy, emaciated cow was found tethered. Her perineal area was heavily soiled and necrotic (Fig. 5.7). The farmer reported that she had had 'a difficult calving'. Checks revealed that the veterinary surgeon had not been contacted regarding this cow. She was euthanased.

Post-mortem examination:

A large (150 × 160 mm) necrotic area involved the anus, rectum, vulva and urethra.

A common entrance to the rectum and vagina had formed and this cloaca-like cavity was heavily contaminated with faeces. The lining was necrotic. The bladder was congested and partially filled with fawn–grey fluid.

The post-calving uterus showed well formed caruncles and widespread endometritis.

More generally, the cow was in extremely poor bodily condition, had low-grade parasitism and was suffering from mastitis.

Photography:

Photography of this extensively damaged area was aided by the insertion of coloured markers in the rectum, vagina and urethra before dissection. After the damaged organs had been opened, the coloured markers were replaced and further photographs taken. This process created a series of photographs that clearly demonstrated the location of the various structures and allowed the Court to appreciate the extent of the damage (Fig. 5.8).

The issues:

This is a straightforward case of neglect following calving. However, there are three levels of neglect here. The initial one concerns the gross mal-handling of the cow, during calving, that resulted in the perineal, vaginal and anal damage. Secondly, no immediate veterinary treatment was sought or given. Thirdly, chronic neglect resulted in extensive necrosis and unnecessary suffering associated with the untreated tears and the subsequent infections in the urinary bladder and uterus. The forensic report needs to reflect these different and additive insults.

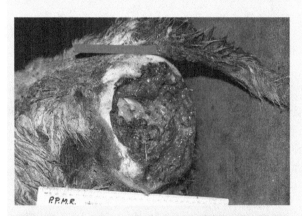

Fig. 5.7 – Cow. Necrosis and heavy faecal soiling of the perineum resulting from damage sustained during an assisted calving. No veterinary attention or treatment had been sought.

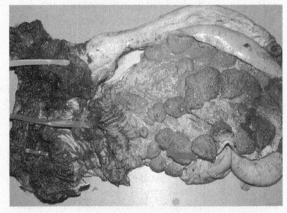

Fig. 5.8 – Cow (see Fig. 5.7). For clarity of description of the injuries, coloured coded markers were used to highlight the entrances to the anus/rectum (green), vagina (red) and bladder (blue).

Case study 5.3: Neglect of forelimb of dog following a road accident

Clinical history:

'Billy' suffered serious injury to the motor and sensory nerve supply to the right forelimb when involved in a road accident. The owner failed to return Billy for veterinary examination and failed to take adequate care of the leg over the following 12 months. The limb became infected and necrotic, resulting in the animal's collapse. Veterinary treatment was not sought. The owner crudely amputated the lower part of the limb and staunched the blood flow with a hot iron. The stump of bones and muscle remained uncovered until the dog was taken into care and treated surgically.

Post-mortem examination:

Two portions of limb were examined: the decomposing lower end of the limb that had been cut off by the owner and discarded in the garden, and the part amputated by the veterinary surgeon. These specimens were radiographed, photographed and dissected.

Case study 5.3: Neglect of forelimb of dog following a road accident (*continued*)

The foot showed the characteristic injuries associated with chronic excoriation of the top of the foot (Fig. 5.9). Loss of some of the phalanges accompanied by abrasion of the metacarpals and tendons highlighted the long-standing nature of the injuries.

New bone formation above, but not below, the point where the owner had severed the leg confirmed that the lower part of the leg had been removed several weeks before Billy was taken into care. Remodelling of the stump had occurred following the 'operation' by the owner.

The issues:

Billy failed to receive adequate care and attention in the period following the road accident.

In addition, forensic examination demonstrated neglect at various stages in the subsequent months:

- Long-term neglect (for approximately 12 months) that resulted in infection and necrosis in the lower limb and contributed to the collapse of the dog
- The crude method used to sever the limb through viable tissue
- The open, raw stump caused by severance of the limb
- The absence of evidence of veterinary treatment.

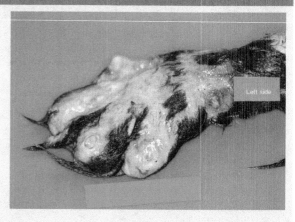

Fig. 5.9 – Upper aspect of the right forepaw of a dog showing damage caused by chronic excoriation and infection.

Case study 5.4: Neglect of injury to jaw of Yorkshire terrier

Clinical history:

An elderly man made an appointment at the veterinary clinic for euthanasia of his Yorkshire terrier. When presented, the veterinary surgeon noticed that the left eye appeared to be missing and that the lower jaw was also absent. The dog was dirty and in very poor bodily condition. On questioning, the owner offered no adequate explanation for the changes to the eye and admitted that he did not seek veterinary attention for this injury. Regarding the jaw, he claimed that the dog's teeth were missing but could shed no further light on when, or how, the jaw was lost. He, again, agreed that he had not taken the dog for veterinary examination for this problem. The owner stated that he had tried to feed the dog but that he could cope no longer.

Post-mortem examination:

This little dog was emaciated and faeces were adherent to the perineum. The left eye was collapsed. The stomach contained a small quantity of food.

Radiography showed absence of all teeth. Approximately half the length of both right and left sides of the lower jaw bones (extending from the midpoint to the point of the jaw) was absent. There was no radiological evidence of infection in the remaining portions of the lower jaw. The premaxilla (which forms part of the upper jaw) was also absent.

Dissection revealed that the truncated ends of the lower jaw were covered with connective tissue, confirming that the bone had been missing for a period of weeks. As there was no effective floor to the mouth beyond the truncated jaw, the tongue hung down through the gap (Fig. 5.10).

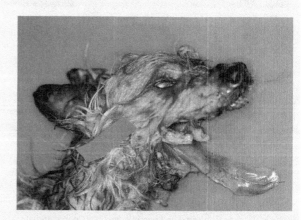

Fig. 5.10 – Dog. Loss of the forward (rostral) portions of both lower jaw bones. The nature of the initial injuries remained obscure. Gross neglect had occurred over an extended period. No veterinary attention had been sought.

Case study 5.4: Neglect of injury to jaw of Yorkshire terrier (*continued*)

The issues:

Forensic examination was requested to establish the precise nature of the bizarre changes to the jaw. Although the sequence of events that led to loss of the jawbone could not be ascertained with any degree of confidence, pathology clarified the timescale (many weeks) required for the bone to be removed and for the ends of the damaged jaw to be encased in connective tissue. It

was established that there had been no surgery to the jaw. Statements were also made regarding the suffering related to the original injury that caused the necrosis and loss of the jawbone. Additionally, informed comment was made on the relationship between the jaw problems, the resulting difficulty in eating and drinking, and the lack of other chronic systemic disease to account for the emaciation.

Case study 5.5: Neglect of ingrowing horn

Clinical history:

A member of the public reported that the horns of a bull appeared to have grown round into the sides of the bull's face (Fig. 5.11). Animal welfare officers and the police attended the farm, but the owner was unable to catch or control the bull. A marksman killed the bull with a shot to the head. Darkness was descending by this time and the dead animal was left in the field. In the morning when the authorities arrived at the farm it was noticed that the ends of the horns had been sawn off. The owner

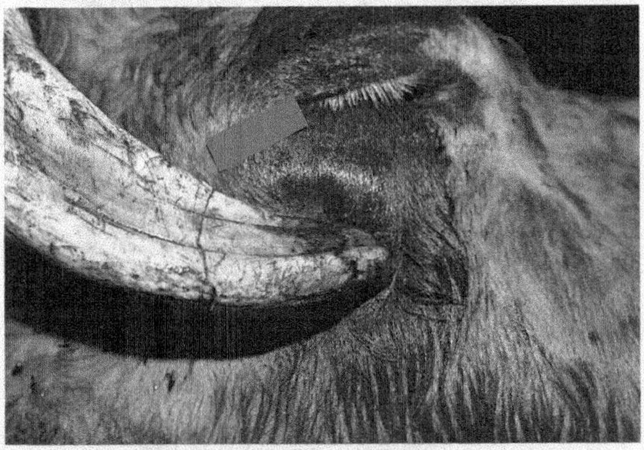

Fig. 5.11 – Bull. Curved horn pressing into the skin on the right side of the face. Note the line across the horn towards the tip where the horn tip had been cut off post mortem.

admitted that she was responsible. The police recovered two portions of horn believed to be the portions that had been cut off during the night. The head and pieces of horn were submitted for forensic examination.

Post-mortem examination:

The horns curved forwards, downwards and inwards towards the head below and behind the eyes. The portions of horn recovered by the police made exact physical matches with the cut ends of the horns, and aligned with and pressed into damaged skin and underlying tissues on the sides of the bull's head.

The skin, particularly on the left side, was grossly thickened and a hole 28 mm in diameter penetrated through the skin. The tip of the horn pressed against the zygomatic arch behind the eye. Straight vertical incisions extending above and below the skin hole had been made post mortem. The skin on the right side of the head was similarly thickened and calloused, but was depressed rather than penetrated.

The issues:

The primary issue was whether the bull had suffered as the horns grew into the face. Gross pathology and histopathology demonstrated long-standing changes to the skin, muscle and connective tissue, scar tissue formation in the depths of the hole, and the presence of infection in the hole on the left side of the face. Similar but less severe changes affected the right side. There was agreement that unnecessary suffering had been caused by neglect of these injuries.

Case study 5.5: Neglect of ingrowing horn (*continued*)

The investigation raised several other forensic questions. First, were the portions of horn (found by the police) definitely those that had been sawn off during the night? Achieving *exact physical fits* between the cut ends of the horn and the recovered pieces of horn was extremely persuasive that these were, indeed, the missing horn tips. The additional questions concerned the incised wounds extending above and below the hole of the left side of the face. What caused these marks? When had they occurred? Did they confound the examination of the original wound?

The wounds were incised wounds caused by a sharp blade (Fig. 5.12). As there was no evidence of bleeding, exudation of serum, scab formation or healing associated with these cuts, it was concluded that they were inflicted after death. These cuts were described in the pathology report, but, as they were clearly separate from, and did not obscure, the chronic pathological changes in the skin, they did not complicate the interpretation of the primary lesions.

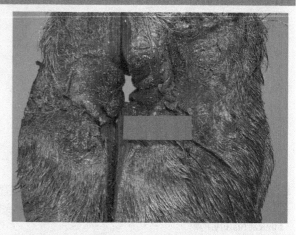

Fig. 5.12 – Bull (see Fig. 5.11). Skin from left side of face showing (a) the central hole caused by the tip of the horn and (b) post-mortem incised wounds above and below the hole.

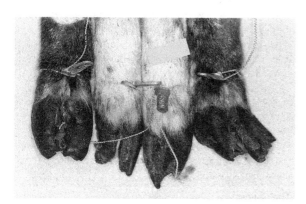

Fig. 5.13 – Feet of sheep, with identity seals on each foot.

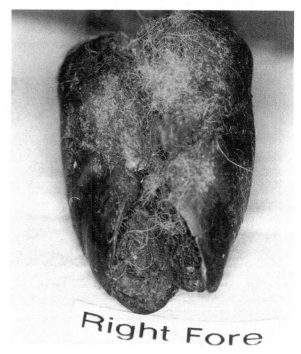

Fig. 5.14 – Sheep's foot as first presented, showing overgrowth of horn and sole obscured by wool and faeces.

or other identification of the animal that leaves no doubt about the origin of the specimen (Fig. 5.13). The label, or associated paperwork, should also specifically identify which leg or foot is being submitted. Much pathology time can be wasted deciding whether the portion of lower limb is from the right or left side or from the fore or hind limbs.

The following simple procedure for handling the samples has proved its worth:

- The specimens are photographed in the state in which they arrive, frequently heavily soiled with a mixture of faeces, straw and earth (Fig. 5.14).
- The legs and feet are washed in lukewarm water and careful note is made of any evidence of treatments (e.g. copper sulphate or purple sprays) on the skin and horn (Fig. 5.15).

- Once cleaned, the limbs are re-photographed to show conformation, external lesions and overgrowth of horn, etc. (Figs 5.16 & 5.17).
- If fractures or chronic infection are suspected, the limb is radiographed.

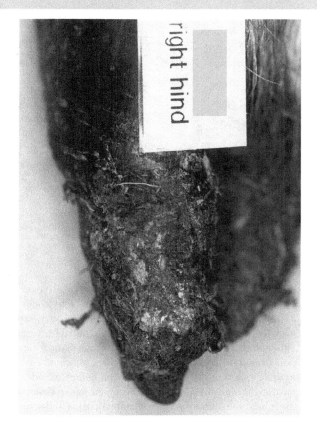

Fig. 5.15 – Sheep's foot with traces of copper sulphate treatment on the hoof horn.

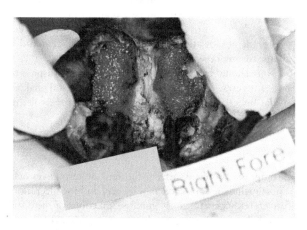

Fig. 5.16 – Sheep's foot (see Fig. 5.14). After washing, the extent of the sole ulceration can be appreciated.

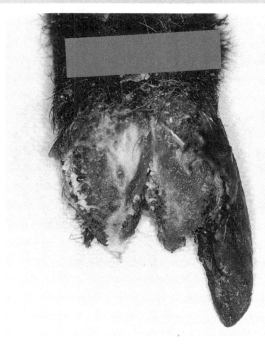

Fig. 5.17 – One of 26 feet from a batch of sheep transported to market. This foot was balled up with faeces when first examined.

- 'Cleaned bone' preparations are readily prepared by removal (by dissection) of the majority of the soft tissues followed by digestion in a solution of biological washing powder at 60°C. This is a rather imprecise process involving 'one or two scoops of biological washing powder in a water bath or bucket'. Regular examination of the specimens will ensure that the process is not allowed to progress to the stage of damaging the outer surface of the bone. Care needs to be taken with sub-adult bones where the enzymes in the solution may cause excessive damage. An alternative method is the use of washing soda at 65–70°C. Again, the strength and duration of treatment is gauged by experience and regular observations.
- In cases of suspected laminitis, removal of the hoof horn[8] aids the investigation.
- The affected hoof and lower limb is sectioned, by saw, sagittally or through the midline.

A common defence against alleged neglect of lame farm animals is that the animal 'was in good bodily condition – was putting on weight' and therefore could not have been suffering. This is not supported by observation of injured animals. Many farm animals with long-standing, painful conditions such as untreated limb factures, chronic septic conditions in their feet or osteoarthritis remain in fair to good bodily condition. It is incumbent on the veterinarian to advise the court that the contention that 'an animal in good condition cannot be in significant pain' is unsubstantiated and should be rejected.

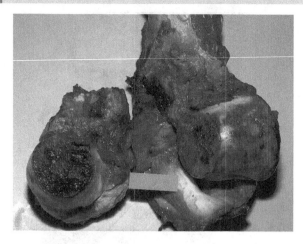

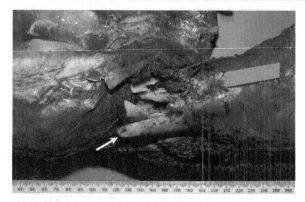

Fig. 5.19 – Cow. Compound comminuted fracture of metacarpus showing rounded ends of bone fragments (arrow) and necrotic, infected soft tissues around the fracture site.

Fig. 5.18 – Cow noted to be lame on arrival at market. Recent fracture of femur (less than 12 hours old) showing clotting of blood but no evidence of repair or infection.

Fractures

The central issues in fracture cases are, first, when did the fracture occur and, secondly, was veterinary advice and treatment sought?

Recent fractures are characterised by fresh haemorrhage around the fracture site and adjacent soft tissues, clot formation between the fractured pieces, fibrin strands over and between the fractured ends of the bone, and absence of obvious repair (Fig. 5.18).

Accumulation of yellow, serum-like fluid around the site or in the soft tissues distal to the fracture suggests that haematoma retraction has occurred to some extent; this indicates a longer post-traumatic period.

Periosteal proliferation, which is the first step in external callus formation, may begin within 24 hours of fracture, but this response is not visible macroscopically at that stage. Early mineralisation of the callus may develop within 1 week of injury, although radiographic evidence of mineralisation is unlikely to be seen until 2 weeks post-trauma.

Older fractures have callus formation. Where there has been minimal movement at the fracture site, callus formation can be relatively modest. However, in many farm animal cases, obvious callus formation results from gross displacement of the fractured ends, or lack of adequate immobilisation of the fracture.

The most common fractures in cattle involve the metacarpal or metatarsal bones.[9] Frequently, these fractures are comminuted, and they may be open or closed. Neglect of closed metacarpal or metatarsal fractures results in damage to the overlying skin as the animal attempts to bear weight on the damaged leg. The situation progresses to heavy contamination of the fracture site with suppuration and necrosis of soft tissues and bone. In comminuted fractures, fragments of devitalised bone may be present and the margins of the bony fragments may be worn by prolonged or frequent movement against one another or by contact with the ground (Fig. 5.19). Callus formation may not occur in these heavily contaminated comminuted fractures, although there will be some attempts at scar tissue formation around the site. Obvious haemorrhage may not be seen in these long-standing cases, but histopathology may demonstrate haemosiderin in the fibrous repair tissue. Distal to the injury, the limb may be swollen by oedema and serum leakage.

Closed fractures of long bones (e.g. radius and ulna) may also become infected if left untreated. Such injuries may result in non-union at the fracture site, abscess formation, destruction of bone and new bone formation on the periosteal surfaces of adjacent viable bone (Fig. 5.20). Eventually, the abscessation may track to the surface and discharge through the skin.

Note should be taken of factors that may predispose to bone fractures. An example is fracture of the distal phalanx (pedal bone) where infection extending from the sole, or old age changes to the bone, may be involved.

Foot lameness

A range of problems affects the feet of farm livestock. These include lesions such as sole, heel and toe ulceration, foreign body penetration, laminitis, infections of the distal interphalangeal joint, generalised sepsis within the deeper tissues of the foot, interdigital pathology, wall defects and malformations.

Forensic examination attempts to define the duration of these changes and to reveal whether or not appropriate treatment was given (e.g. amputation of toe in cases of pedal joint sepsis). Radiography can be very helpful in these chronic cases (Fig. 5.21). The presence of advanced abscessation within the foot, sloughing of hoof horn, infection with maggots, and marked ulceration of the sole or toes provides clear evidence of neglect.

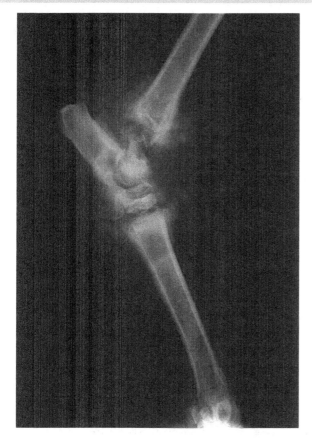

Fig. 5.20 – Sheep. Non-union of fracture at lower end of tibia showing lysis of bone and attempted repair.

Deformities

It is a matter of judgement whether deformities to the limb are, in themselves, a cause of unnecessary suffering. A lamb born with an ankylosed carpus may hobble but may not suffer. However, a lamb with a deformed limb caused by mal-union of an untreated overriding fracture of the humerus would undoubtedly have suffered. The calf with congenital shortening and deformities of the limbs may not have painful limb joints, but the abnormal gait may be causing problems in the spine, resulting in unnecessary pain and distress. A clinician/behaviourist will be able to provide better insights in these cases than a pathologist.

Degenerative conditions

Degenerative joint disease in older animals and osteochrondrosis dissecans in rapidly growing cattle are undoubtedly painful and are manifest by lameness or, for example, reluctance of bulls to mount cows. The lesions include loss or wear of articular cartilage, exposure and eburnation of the underlying bone, and fibrosis around the affected joints (Fig. 5.22). Haemorrhage in the joint cavity, joint capsule or surrounding fibrosis is evidence of recent damage. These lesions should be exposed by dissection.

Miscellaneous trauma and infection

Rope, wire, or chain wrapped around the lower parts of the limbs for restraint, or by accident, can lead to severe injury if neglected. Swelling of the foot and lower end of the leg is accompanied by pressure damage to the skin and underlying soft tissues, leading to an encircling wound that may penetrate to the bone. The extent of swelling, infection and attempted repair by granulation tissue are useful markers when assessing whether the ligature was applied recently or some time ago (Fig. 5.23).

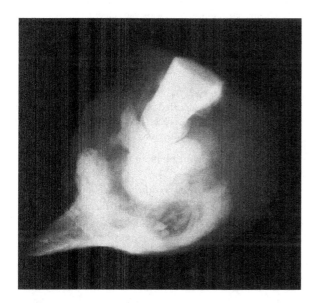

Fig. 5.21 – The owner of this cow claimed that the animal showed no lameness before transportation to market. The radiograph highlights the chronicity and extent of damage to the foot.

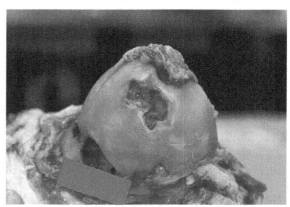

Fig. 5.22 – Two-year-old bull with severe degenerative joint disease of weeks or months in duration.

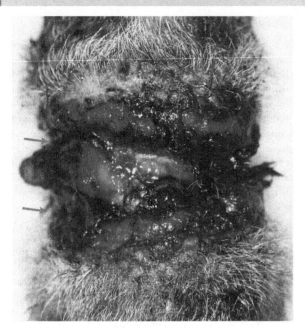

Fig. 5.23 – Cow. Hobbled and neglected leading to pressure damage to skin and underlying tissues. Arrows indicate where the rope had been wound twice around the leg.

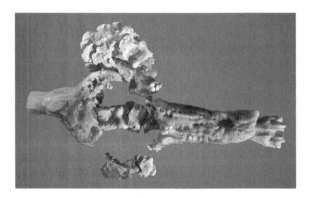

Fig. 5.24 – Goat. Chronic septic arthritis of the hock joint with drainage leading to cellulitis and bony plaque formation over the metatarsus.

Untreated cellulitis related to drainage of infection from a septic focus higher in the limb (e.g. septic arthritis) may, if the overlying skin does not slough, undergo a process of ossification that extends over a period of weeks or months. This gives rise to the formation of irregular bony plaques in the subcutaneous tissues overlying, say, the metacarpus or metatarsus (Fig. 5.24). The periosteal surface of the long bones may be extensively eroded where the bony plaques are in close contact with it.

Natural disease

Natural disease is encountered, to some degree or other, during the course of many forensic examinations. Usually

Case study 5.6: Neglect of fractures and spinal problems

Clinical history:

A 6.5-year-old cross-bred bull terrier living with a violent owner (who had previously been prosecuted for physical abuse of this dog) was seized following reports that she had been physically abused. Multiple deep, scabbed lesions on the head were recorded on first examination at the veterinary clinic. The lips were bruised and sore, and all four canine teeth were broken. Extensive bruising affected the ventral neck and left axilla, whilst subcutaneous emphysema extended from the ventral neck and sternum over the whole of the rib cage. Radiography detected several fractured ribs and lysis of bone in proximal femur and in the lumbar spine. Progressive deterioration in the dog's condition led to euthanasia.

Post-mortem examination:

Multiple myeloma had resulted in 14 pathological rib fractures of various ages, collapse of the last thoracic and first lumbar vertebrae with compression of the spinal cord, tumour masses in the proximal femur and in the small intestine.

The issues:

There was no direct evidence that the rib fractures had been caused by physical violence by the owner. However, it was accepted that early diagnosis and supportive treatment would have guided the management of this progressive natural disease and prevented immense suffering. The owner was convicted of cruelty to animals by failing to provide veterinary treatment.

The healing skin lesions on the head were probably caused by burning (e.g. by a cigarette end), but, although histopathological examination eliminated other disease conditions such as pemphigus, parasitic infections and dermatophytosis, the evidence was inadequate to sustain a further cruelty charge.

it involves middle-aged or older animals. Disease processes should be recorded, reported and interpreted in the light of the circumstances of the case. The forensic report should address disease-related questions such as:

- Did the disease contribute to the poor condition of the animal?
- Is the disease related to other aspects of the case?
- Does the presence of disease alter the interpretation of other post-mortem findings?
- Would it be reasonable to expect the average owner or keeper of the animal to have noticed any signs of ill health?
- Should veterinary treatment have been given?

Such questions are important for two reasons. First, unnecessary suffering may have arisen directly through neglect of the disease process. Case study 5.6 highlights

Case study 5.7

Clinical history:

An elderly dog suffering from untreated hyperadrenocorticism was polydipsic, had begun wetting during the night, was ravenously hungry and his progressive bilateral alopecia and distended abdomen made him unsightly. The owner decided to dispose of the dog by drowning him in the bath and dumping the body in a stream on some rough ground.

Post-mortem examination:

Death by drowning was suspected. Marked, chronic changes in the adrenal glands supported a diagnosis of hyperadrenocorticism.

The issues:

Forensic examination of this dog highlighted two issues. First, death appeared to have resulted from drowning, and this would have entailed significant suffering. Secondly, unnecessary suffering had been caused through lack of veterinary treatment of the adrenal disease.

the relationship between diagnostic and forensic examination. Secondly, the clinical manifestations of the disease may have caused changes in the animal that led to abuse (Case study 5.7).

References

1. Anon. The American Heritage® dictionary of the English language, 4th edn. Boston: Houghton Mifflin; 2000.

2. Scrimshaw NS, Taylor CE, Gordon JE. Interaction of malnutrition and infection. WHO Monograph Series 57. Geneva: World Health Organisation; 1968.

3. Keusch GT. Malnutrition, infection and immune function. In: Suskind RM, Lewinter-Suskind L, eds. The malnourished child. Nestlé Nutrition Workshop Series, 19. New York: Vevey/Raven Press; 1990:37–59.

4. Saunders AB, How SJ, Lloyd DH et al. The effect of energy malnutrition in ruminants on experimental infection with *Dermatophilus congolensis*. J Comp Pathol 1990; 103: 361–368.

5. Blowey R. Cattle lameness and hoofcare: an illustrated guide. Ipswich: Farming Press; 1993.

6. Hirst WH, Le Fevre AM, Logue DN et al. A systematic compilation and classification of the literature on lameness in cattle. Vet J 2002; 164:7–19.

7. Blowey RW, Weaver AD. Color atlas of diseases and disorders of cattle, 2nd edn. London: Mosby; 2003.

8. Ossent P, Lischer CJ. The pathology of digital disease and theories on the pathogenesis of bovine laminitis. Ir Vet J 1996; 49:485–487.

9. Tulleners EP. Metacarpal and metatarsal fractures in cattle. Vet Clin North Am Food Anim Pract 1996; 12:199–209.

6 | Wounds and Injuries

Introduction

A wound is generally considered to be a skin injury, caused by some external force, that may extend to deeper tissues. However, external forces may injure (or wound) deeper tissues without necessarily breaching the skin. Such injuries fall within the definition of 'blunt force injuries'. The common denominator in both types of injury is the 'external force'.

In the initial stages of an investigation the immediate concern of the pathologist is to describe the nature and location of the injuries. How the injuries were inflicted, and whether they were accidental or deliberate, can be considered later. This two-stage process encourages a balanced assessment of the injuries and reduces the likelihood of 'jumping to conclusions' early in the investigation.

Skin injuries can be divided into:

- *Blunt force injuries* – abrasions, bruises (contusions), lacerations (split wounds)
- *Sharp force injuries* – incised wounds (cuts or slashes), stab wounds (puncture or penetrating wounds).

Blunt force injuries to deeper tissues include bruising and laceration of muscles, damage to internal organs, and fractures. Stab wounds, in addition to the skin damage, may also injure deeper organs.

Certain terms are commonly used in human forensic medicine and are understood by lawyers and judges. These include: abrasion, laceration, incised wound, puncture wound and perforating wound. Their correct use in veterinary cases simplifies reports (and verbal explanations in Courts) and makes 'animal' cases more understandable to the legal profession and to juries.

Blunt force injuries

General

Blunt force injuries are more commonly encountered in veterinary medicine than wounding by sharp implements. Feet, fists, hammers, sticks, baseball bats, billiard cues and bricks are some of the many implements used to injure animals. The resulting damage may occasionally reflect the type of object used, but for the most part the injuries identify where the blows struck but not the weapon. Although single blows are encountered, most animals have more than one injury, often widely distributed over the head, body and limbs.

Abrasions

Abrasions are the most superficial of wounds to the skin. When the skin collides tangentially with a rough surface, the outer layers (the keratinised parts) are rubbed off, exposing the more sensitive layers (Fig. 6.1). Remnants of the abraded layers may be found piled up at the edge of the wound.

Frequently, abrasions do not bleed but merely leak tissue fluid. This causes the injury to appear wet at first and then to become darker and drier with time. When the slightly deeper layers of the skin are involved, blood may ooze from damaged dermal papillae and a dark scab may form.

In motor vehicle accidents and falls on to rough surfaces, small fragments of grit may be embedded in the abraded surface. Hair protects the skin from many minor blows that would otherwise cause abrasion of bare skin. In domestic animals it is therefore relatively rare to find the patterned or crush abrasions that in human forensic pathology are valuable because they provide clues to the type of object that struck the skin (e.g. the sole of a shoe).

Bruises (contusions)

Bruises (also known as contusions) result from blunt trauma. Blood leaks from vessels within the skin or from deeper tissues. The size and appearance of bruises can depend on factors such as tissue density and the fragility of blood vessels. Tight fibrous tissue discourages the collection of blood, whereas loose, soft, well vascularised tissues allow blood to pool. When the tissues are stretched or crushed against underlying bone, the extent of the bleeding may be increased. Conversely, the malleable abdominal wall frequently shows little or no evidence of bruising even after an impact sufficient to cause extensive damage to internal organs such as liver or spleen.

Not all bruises are immediately obvious. Hair and skin colour commonly obscure intradermal and subcutaneous bleeding. When it is feasible, clipping/shaving or plucking areas of suspected bruising may be helpful in the live animal (Fig. 6.2), even in very dark-coloured animals such as black Labradors (Fig. 6.3). Clipping/shaving can also be done at the start of the post-mortem examination. In many cases,

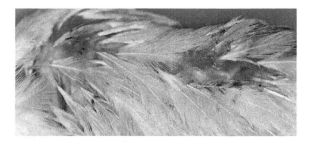

Fig. 6.1 – Domestic hen. Abrasion of the wing showing areas of denudation of the outer layer of skin. The deeper layer of the skin (dermis) is intact.

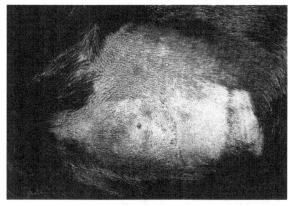

Fig. 6.3 – Labrador. Bruising is less obvious in dark-haired animals than in light-skinned ones. However, clipping the side of the chest of this dog greatly assisted in diagnosing bleeding in the axilla.

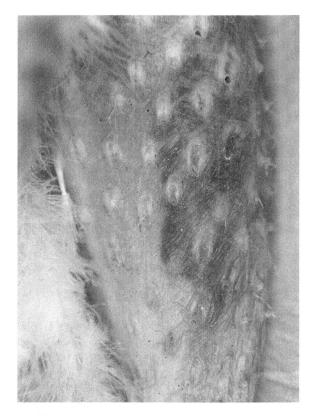

Fig. 6.2 – Domestic hen. Subcutaneous bruising is often obscured by feathers. Plucking of the leg of this hen revealed the extent of the bruising.

however, severe bruising may not be discovered until the skin is reflected at post-mortem examination.

It is good practice to photograph areas of bruising that are found after reflection of the skin *as soon as practicable*. Delay results in the exposed bruise fading, spreading and becoming less clearly defined. There is also a danger that leakage of blood from severed vessels or from body cavities may contaminate the area and confuse the picture.

The margins of bruises spread and blur with time, making the shape of a bruise an unreliable guide to the outline of the object that struck the body. However, blows by sticks, broom handles or similar narrow objects to relatively hairless skin may leave characteristic 'tramline bruises'.[1] The skin along the line of impact is depressed and compressed by the force of the weapon, whereas the skin at the margins of this area is stretched. This action results in the blood vessels at the centre of the injury being compressed whilst those along the margins are torn. As blood flows back into the area, leakage from the torn vessels results in two linear bruises at the margins of the area of contact by the stick.

Stick marks and other bruising related to transport are common in livestock sent for slaughter.[2] They may be recognised in light-skinned pigs before slaughter, but in cattle are more commonly found after skinning. In the subcutis and superficial muscles, the bruises do not usually develop a 'tramline' appearance.

Extensive bruising of livestock, found at slaughter, can be the first direct evidence that a significant husbandry problem exists on a farm (Fig. 6.4) or that there are major deficiencies in the transport arrangements. The veterinarian's report will be a key element in the subsequent investigation.

Age of bruising

As the bruise ages, red cells rupture and haemoglobin degrades. This causes the sequence of colour changes readily seen in animals and birds with light-coloured skin that survive the injury by several days. Observations of poultry[3] record bruises changing from red at 2 minutes post-trauma through dark red–purple at 12 hours, light green–purple at 24 hours, yellow–green–purple by 36 hours, becoming yellow–green at 48 hours and yellow–orange at 72 hours, reducing to be 'slightly yellow' at 96 hours and normal by 120 hours post-injury.

Because of economic losses related to trimming of bruised meat from slaughtered animals, there has been

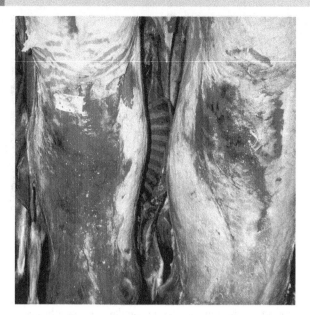

Fig. 6.4 – Deer. A group of abattoir-slaughtered farmed deer showed extensive bruising over their bodies and head. Investigation revealed major problems with on-farm handling of the deer. (By kind permission of Leonard 'Sam' Mansley.)

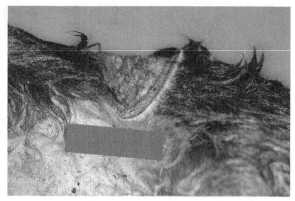

Fig. 6.5 – Dog. Laceration of the skin over the back and on to the flank of a dog killed in a road accident.

considerable interest in establishing when these bruises occurred. The approximate age of bruises in cattle and sheep, as judged by their macroscopic appearance, ranges from red and haemorrhagic between 0 and 10 hours after injury, dark coloured when approximately 24 hours old, watery in consistency by 24–38 hours, and having a rusty orange colour and a soapy texture when more than 3 days.[4]

Research conducted in Australia on lambs and calves[5] has provided a guide to histological ageing of bruising over the 0–48-hour period after trauma in these animals. This research showed that trauma occurring immediately before death can lead to haemorrhage in subcutaneous tissues, in the muscle septa, and between muscle fibres. Small numbers of neutrophils and macrophages are present in the extravasated blood. At 8 hours after trauma, the extent of the bleeding is greater and fibrin strands are recognisable. Many neutrophils and few macrophages are present in the extravasated blood, the damaged muscle and the subcutis. The amount of haemorrhage changes little between 8 and 24 hours after injury, but the ratio of neutrophils and macrophages alters so that they are found in approximately similar numbers at 24 hours. This change in cell population continues over the subsequent 24-hour period, resulting in macrophages greatly outnumbering neutrophils by 48 hours after trauma. At this time, capillaries with plump endothelium can also be seen invading the damaged tissues.

There is a paucity of information on the ageing of bruises in other species. Perhaps the guidelines for lamb and calf bruising are relevant to a range of other animals, but present knowledge is limited and caution is advised when interpreting tissue injury based on observations made in substantially different species.

Haemosiderin deposits are readily identified by the Prussian Blue reaction in macrophages 48 hours after injury. Haemosiderin deposited or trapped in scar tissue may be demonstrated many weeks after injury and may provide convincing evidence of previous bruising in suspected cases of repetitive injury.

Testing for the formation of bilirubin (as haemoglobin is broken down in the area of the bruise) has also been used to estimate the time elapsed since injury. This method is based on the colour change seen in samples of bruised muscle after being soaked in a mixture of trichloroacetic acid and ferric chloride.[4]

Force required to cause bruising

'How much force is required to cause a bruise?' is a frequently asked question to which there is no precise answer. It is often assumed that small bruises correlate with limited force and that larger ones signify impacts of greater force. However, because of the variables noted in the section on bruising (e.g. tissue density and vessel fragility) and other unknown factors, including the bleeding time and the protection offered by coat hair, such assumptions can be misleading. Nevertheless, it is reasonable to conclude that bruising in *deeper* tissues may have required greater force than that resulting in only subcutaneous bruising at a similar site.

Lacerations

Lacerations are caused by blunt trauma that results in tearing or splitting of the tissues. They can be accidental, as in motor vehicle accidents (Fig. 6.5), or can be caused by heavy blows from a blunt weapon, or by violent shaking and tearing, during which the skin and deeper tissues are stretched until they tear.

Lacerations frequently *do not* conform to the shape of the object that inflicted the damage, and severely lacerated muscle may be present underneath *intact* skin (e.g. see Bite wounds).

The margins of lacerated skin wounds are usually irregular and may show abrasion and bruising. Strands of tougher tissue, such as blood vessels, may be seen extending from side to side across the deeper parts of the wound. Bleeding commonly accompanies laceration but the stretching and crushing action of the injury can cause blood vessels to retract, so that the extent of haemorrhage is commonly less than might be expected for the severity of the damage.

Head, face and neck injuries

Head injuries

The head is a common target for blows to dogs and cats. A hammer, stick or spade may be used to club dogs and foxes, whilst hammer blows can also cause fatal head injuries to calves. Whenever possible, the suspect weapon should be examined in order to gauge whether, because of its shape, size and weight, it could have caused the injuries. Equally importantly, it may be found that the flimsiness of the putative weapon raises doubts that it was used to fracture a mature skull. The weapon should be examined for blood traces and adherent hairs (Fig. 6.6).

Small creatures, such as kittens, may suffer major head injury as a result of being held by the hind limbs and swung against a wall or floor. The injuries in these cases are frequently disproportionately severe and cast doubt on the veracity of histories that claim the injuries were the consequence of a 'fall'.

Depending on the type of object striking the head, superficial soft tissue injury might consist of abrasions, lacerations or incised wounds. Subcutaneous bruising usually accompanies blunt trauma to the head and can be valuable in establishing the nature and direction of the blow(s) (Case study 6.1, Fig. 6.7). Extensive or marked intramuscular

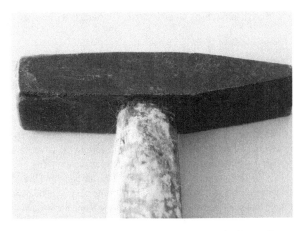

Fig. 6.6 – Hammer used in a sustained attack on an elderly dog. Note blood and hairs on shaft and head of hammer.

Case study 6.1

Clinical history:

A 4-month-old mongrel puppy was recovered from a rubbish pile following a domestic dispute during which the female partner fled in fear of her life.

Post-mortem examination:

The only external sign of injury was a small bruise on the left side of the head, at the base of the ear. Internally, severe bruising was present over the right dorsal and lateral aspect of the head but the skull was not fractured in this area (Fig. 6.7). On the left side of the face and head, bruising overlay part of the upper jaw and cheekbone, and extended into the adjacent muscles. The cheekbone was fractured in two places and a depressed fracture involved much of the side of the skull. A large haemorrhage was present within the left side of the brain.

The issues:

1 How many blows were struck?

The areas of injury were well defined in this case and guidance on the number of times that the puppy was struck was important. The nature and distribution of the bruising and fractures suggested one or more blows to the left side of the

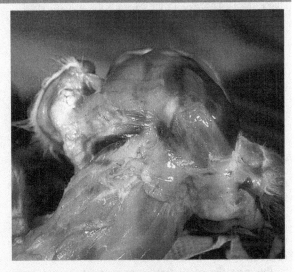

Fig. 6.7 – Puppy. Extensive haemorrhage over the back of the head on the right side. The skull was not fractured at this site. Note the line of haemorrhage along back of skull from base of left ear, probably caused by sudden over-flexion of neck when head was struck.

Case study 6.1 (continued)

head with a further heavy blow to the top of the right side of the head.

2 What type of object or weapon was used?

Nothing could be stated with certainty about the object or weapon that caused the damage in this particular case, but kicking or punching can result in this type of injury in puppies or kittens.

3 Was suffering caused?

Death resulted from haemorrhage within the brain. However, such haemorrhage takes time to develop and there was no

basis to suppose that death was instantaneous or that the puppy was insensible throughout the period when blood was leaking into the brain. It was considered highly likely, therefore, that the puppy suffered (a) during the actual assault when the cheekbone and skull were fractured and (b) during the subsequent period of bleeding into the brain.

Case study 6.2

Clinical history:

A bull terrier-type dog was exhumed from a flowerbed after information was received that she had been beaten to death. The owner said that the dog had died from a 'heart attack'. Later he changed the story, claiming that he had hit her, lightly, with a baseball bat after she had defaecated on the furniture and the children's clothes. The owner claimed that he hit her on the head and that she lay down in the living room. He found her dead in that room some time afterwards.

Post-mortem examination:

The dog, which had been buried for approximately 4 weeks, showed advanced post-mortem change but was in reasonable bodily condition. There were no skeletal fractures and no evidence of head injury. However, extensive bruising affected the back, chest (both sides) and the left side of the abdominal wall. Semi-solid material, which was considered to have leaked from the stomach or small bowel, was free within the abdominal cavity. No other significant injuries were present.

The issues:

1 Was the degree of post-mortem change an impediment to the investigation?

Advancing post-mortem decomposition obscures the finer details of changes that occurred before death – small bruises,

for example, become less distinct. In addition, post-mortem leakage of blood pigments from blood vessels may mimic small bruises. However, in this case, there was obvious bruising on the body related to significant blunt trauma to the chest and abdomen.

Post-mortem changes introduced some uncertainty with regard to the final cause of death inasmuch as rupture of the stomach/intestines could have occurred after death. It was absence of other significant pathological changes to account for the death of this dog that suggested that leakage of gut contents into the abdominal cavity was an ante-mortem event. Lack of immediate veterinary attention for such a catastrophic event would have resulted in shock and death.

2 Was there evidence of diarrhoea to account for the history of inappropriate elimination in the house?

Forming faeces in the colon were of normal consistency and colour, suggesting that the explanation given by the owner for his outburst of rage was false.

3 Was there evidence of head injury that might have rendered the dog insensible?

No head injuries were present and this finding, again, cast doubt on the owner's story.

haemorrhage in the temporalis muscles of dogs suggests high-energy trauma.

Absence of bruising over the head in cases where there is a history (or witness evidence) of the animal having been beaten on the head, suggests that either the history is wrong (Case study 6.2) or the beating occurred after death.

Interpretation of bilaterally symmetrical areas of 'bruising' on the skull needs to be approached with caution. Usually these marks are normal anatomical features that are generally overlooked in diagnostic necropsies or they are post-mortem artefacts.

Skull fractures and specific injuries

Radiological interpretation

The radiological classification used for skull fractures in abused children[6] is equally appropriate for abused pets and livestock. Skull fractures are divided into simple or complex categories. Simple fractures are single lines that extend in a straight, jagged or curved manner. These fractures do not cross sutures. In complex fractures there is more than one fracture line. Further useful descriptors are comminuted, depressed and elevated.

Parietal crest

Because of the prominence and strength of the parietal crest in adult badgers, dogs and pigs, fracture of this crest suggests a direct heavy blow to the top of the head (Case study 6.3, Fig. 6.8).

Depressed fractures

Complex depressed fracture of the skull often can be readily identified on X-ray. However, the extent of the damage is sometimes easier to appreciate at post-mortem examination (Case study 6.4, Figs 6.9 & 6.10).

Depressed fractures over the frontal bones and those involving the frontal sinuses are sometimes less obvious on X-ray than fractures of the cranial vault. Compression of the brain can occur beneath the depressed bone but the brain substance is not necessarily lacerated or penetrated.

Hammer attack

Hammer attacks can cause depressed skull fractures and these may be more common over the frontal sinuses than elsewhere. There may be marked haemorrhage into one or

---

Case study 6.3

Clinical history:

An adult female badger was found dead in a small stream.

Post-mortem examination:

Three small superficial wounds were present on the head. Reflection of the skin from the head revealed massive haemorrhage over the top of the head and extending down across the forehead. Linear laceration of the muscles was present midline on the head parallel to the parietal crest. This crest was fractured with two large portions being displaced (Fig. 6.8). No other skull fractures were detected. Intramuscular haemorrhage was found to extend down the right side of the head. Haemorrhage was present on the undersurface of the brainstem and in the sulci of the cerebrum.

The cause of death was drowning.

The issues:

The locus where the badger was found was distant from a road. There were no fractures of leg bones or spine to suggest a motor vehicle accident. Yet, the substantial parietal crest on the

skull was fractured in two places. The most probable cause of this type of injury is a heavy blow. It was suspected that this badger was the victim of a deliberate attack and had been struck on the head by a heavy weapon. Whether the badger was then placed in the stream, or had fallen into the water whilst stunned, could not be determined.

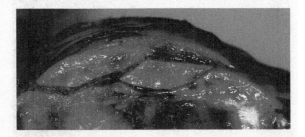

Fig. 6.8 – Badger. Fractures of the parietal crest caused by a heavy blow to the top of the head.

Case study 6.4

Clinical history:

A terrier-type bitch, aged between 5 and 7 months, was reportedly struck on the head by the owner's husband with the handle of his walking stick. X-ray plates showed complex fracturing of the top of the skull and, in view of the severity of the injuries (Fig. 6.9), the dog was euthanased.

Post-mortem examination:

Post-mortem examination revealed the full extent and distribution of the cranial fractures (Fig. 6.10). Additionally, bruising was present over the ribs, although no rib fractures were found and no significant injury affected the heart or lungs.

The issues:

The clinical history indicated that the dog was struck only once but the post-mortem findings raised doubts over this version of

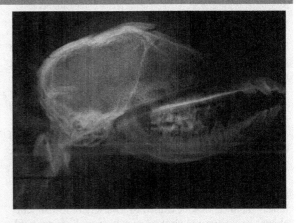

Fig. 6.9 – Puppy. Radiograph of skull showing multiple fractures.

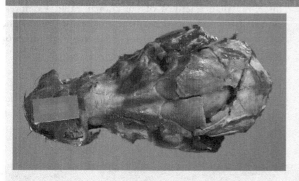

events. The position and shape of the skull injury correlated well with the history that it was the handle of a walking stick that struck the dog's head. However, whether it was a single blow (or several blows) that caused the severe damage to the skull could not be determined, but the bruising over the ribs indicated that the attack had also involved striking the dog around the body. Regarding the question of suffering, it was clear that this young dog had suffered enormously from the head injuries, which were not immediately fatal, the dog being semi-conscious when examined. The suffering may, indeed, have begun before the head injury when she was struck about the body.

Fig. 6.10 – Puppy (as in Fig. 6.9). Extent of skull injury is more readily appreciated following reflection of soft tissues.

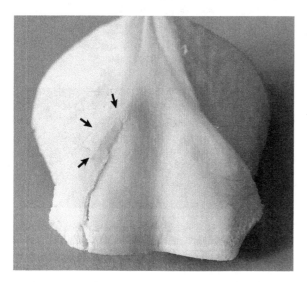

Fig. 6.11 – Adult dog. Struck on forehead with hammer. In addition to the linear fracture, note the adjacent fine fractures (arrows) in the outer bone plate. These give an indication of the profile of the hammer head.

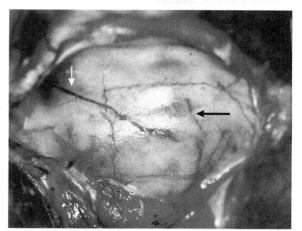

Fig. 6.12 – Cat. Struck on head by a relatively heavy bladed knife. Note cut in frontal bones (white arrow) above right eye leading to linear fracture of left parietal bone. A second fracture (black arrow) of parietal bone was caused by a separate blow.

both of the frontal sinuses. The shape of the depressed area may not, however, accurately replicate the outline of the hammer head, although it may give some indication of the size of the hammer head. Other attacks may result in what at first sight appear to be simple linear fractures, but careful examination of the cleaned skull under good lighting may reveal additional fine cracks in the outer plate of the bone, giving a better indication of the weapon's profile (Fig. 6.11).

Linear fractures

Linear fractures may be caused by a variety of instruments, objects or circumstances. Separate fracture lines probably indicate separate blows (Fig. 6.12).

Crushed skull

Deliberate (Fig. 6.13) or accidental crushing of the skull may look similar on initial examination. Major distortion of the shape of the head is accompanied by haemorrhage from the mouth, nose and ears. If the skin is lacerated, neural tissue may exude from the wounds. However, there may be other injuries that suggest a motor vehicle accident or witness evidence pointing to non-accidental injury.

Suture separation (diastasis)

Forceful impact on the head of a young animal may result in well defined bruising over frontal bones, other bony prominences and along the mandibles. However, no fractures may be found in these areas. Nevertheless, the force of the blow and the resulting distortion of the cranium may

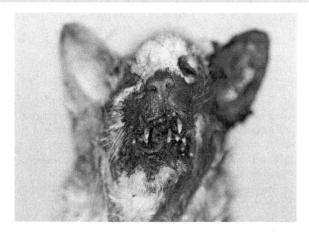

Fig. 6.13 – Cat. Head crushed between a brick and the kerbstone.

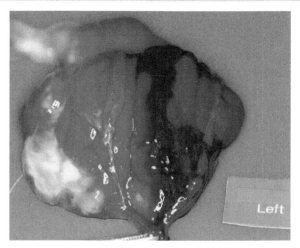

Fig. 6.15 – Cat. The dura mater has been reflected to show an extensive subdural haemorrhage over the left side of the brain.

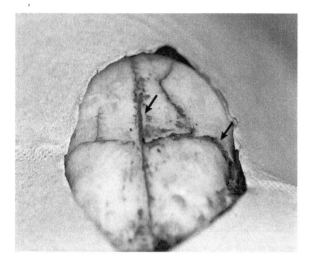

Fig. 6.14 – Cat. Linear fractures of the parietal bones are accompanied by diastasis (arrows) of sutures between the left parietal and left frontal bones and the right parietal bone.

give rise to separation (diastasis) of suture lines (Fig. 6.14). 'Springing' of sutures may affect the vault or floor of the cranium. If these diastases are bilaterally symmetrical on X-ray, they can be dismissed as normal anatomical features, but careful scrutiny may indicate that separation occurred following distortion of the normal shape of the head. Fracture or diastasis in the floor of the cranium can lead to considerable bleeding from the nose as blood tracks forward into the nasal cavities.

Intracranial haemorrhage

Three types of intracranial haemorrhage are recognised:

1. *Extradural* haemorrhage forms in the potential space between the skull and the dura mater. It usually follows fracture of the skull and rupture of a meningeal artery.

2. *Subdural* haemorrhage is *always* due to trauma and arises after tearing of the communicating veins (Fig. 6.15). It is unlikely that the actual bleeding points will be found and it is important to recognise that the blood may flow some distance from the original site. In veterinary medicine, most cases of subdural haemorrhage are found associated with substantial head injury, but skull fracture is not a requirement.

3. *Subarachnoid* haemorrhage occurs in all penetrating injuries of the brain. Many trauma cases with *extradural* and *subdural* haemorrhage will also show *subarachnoid* haemorrhage. *Subarachnoid* haemorrhage mixes with the cerebrospinal fluid and this makes it less likely to clot and therefore more mobile, allowing it to flow, unclotted, away from the injury. In human beings, shearing forces that tear the bridging veins may cause *subarachnoid* haemorrhage.[7] Similar events are yet to be established in veterinary medicine.

Facial injuries including fracture of the cheekbone (zygomatic arch)

Generally, the bones overlying the nose are less robust and less well protected than those over the main part of the skull. Consequently, weapons and blows that would inflict only superficial soft tissue damage over the top of the head can result in extensive fracturing of the face (Case study 6.5, Fig. 6.16).

Fracture of the cheekbone (zygomatic arch), if caused by ante-mortem trauma to the side of the face/head, is accompanied by local haemorrhage and bruising, as in Case study 6.1. However, the junction between the zygomatic processes of the zygomatic and malar bones occasionally remains open in adult dogs and has the potential to be

Clinical history:

The police were informed of two men beating someone, or some animal, on an area of waste ground. The body of an adult mongrel bitch was recovered and taken to a veterinary surgeon for examination. An incomplete post-mortem examination was performed at the veterinary surgery and the cause of death was not established. The body was referred for further examination. Investigations by the police and animal welfare inspectors discovered that she was 7 years old and that she may have been beaten with a billiard cue.

Post-mortem examination:

Various post-mortem incisions had been made in the skin of the head, back and abdomen by the veterinary surgeon. The body cavities had been opened and small samples of various internal organs had been taken, but the organs had not been removed for full examination. The incisions to the abdomen and chest had been sutured.

The referral post-mortem examination revealed multiple injuries to the bones of nose, face, roof of the mouth and floor of the skull (Fig. 6.16). The top of the skull was not fractured, although there was widespread bruising over the top of the head. Death was caused by choking following obstruction of the air passages in the nose and back of the mouth. The obstruction resulted from a combination of collapse of the nose and facial bones and massive bleeding. Recent injuries to the first cervical vertebra, the lumbar spine and chest were also present. An area of older bruising was found on the left side of the chest.

The issues:

The first issue to be addressed was the effect, if any, that the initial 'post-mortem examination' might have on the collection of evidence related to the injuries and death of this dog. This first examination was entirely unskilled, haphazard and inappropriate.

Fortunately, the superficiality of the first examination did not disturb the significant lesions in the head, neck and spine. Consequently, the manner of death was not obscured.

The facial and nasal bones that were fractured during this attack were relatively fragile compared to the sturdy construction of the top of the skull, and this pattern of injury was consistent with the history that she had been beaten with a relatively lightweight weapon (billiard cue). Multiple blows would have been required.

The presence of older bruising over the chest raised the possibility of repetitive injury.

Severe suffering was involved in this case. She was not rendered insensible by the blows to the head but remained conscious until the final stages of asphyxiation.

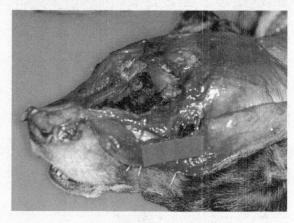

Fig. 6.16 – Adult dog. Multiple injuries to the bones of the nose, face, frontal sinuses, hard palate and floor of skull caused by beating with a billiard cue.

---

misdiagnosed as zygomatic arch fracture. Bruising is not associated with this anatomical anomaly.

Mouth

Blood in the mouth may arise from local injury or more distant sites such as the nasal sinuses, lungs or stomach, or from fractures of the floor of the skull. Food or other material found in the mouth at post-mortem examination may have been ingested but not swallowed, or may have been regurgitated around the time of death. It is good practice to collect and store this material so that it is available for more detailed examination should that be necessary later in the investigation.

Light or medium-force blows to the face can result in bruising of the inside of the lips, and heavier blows can fracture incisor teeth (Fig. 6.17), mandibles, maxillae and the hard palate. Kicks to the jaw can cause bruising in the

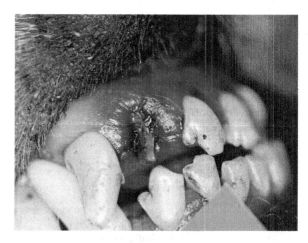

Fig. 6.17 – Adult dog. Recent trauma with fracture of upper incisor.

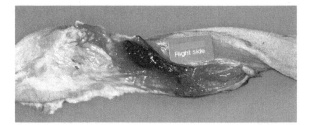

Fig. 6.18 – Puppy. Tongue and pharynx removed to demonstrate haemorrhage in the soft tissue on the medial side of the mandible.

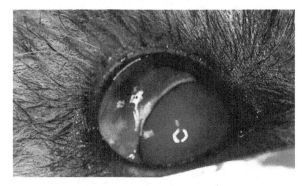

Fig. 6.19 – Adult dog. Conjunctival/scleral haemorrhage. Died from a subdural haemorrhage approximately 24 hours after being beaten over the head and abandoned.

soft tissue on medial aspects of the mandible, and is best seen when the tongue is reflected (Fig. 6.18).

Eyes

Clinicians not uncommonly report subconjunctival[8] and scleral haemorrhages (Fig. 6.19) in dogs and cats suspected of having been beaten around the head, but pathologists note them less frequently. This suggests that these haemorrhages disperse and disappear readily in the early period after death. Nevertheless, the absence of post-mortem evidence of scleral or conjunctival haemorrhage does not negate the ante-mortem clinical observation.

Head trauma can also result in retinal haemorrhage, although natural causes of retinal and vitreous haemorrhage (e.g. severe anaemia or hypertension in cats) need to be considered.[9]

Ears

Examination of ears is usually restricted to the pinnae (ear-flaps) and visible parts of the ear canal. The deeper parts of the ears are rarely examined – perhaps they should be!

Blood on the pinna may arise as a result of local injury, from bleeding elsewhere on the body, or as a consequence of serious head injury with blood issuing along the ear canal.

Chronic inflammatory conditions of the ears may represent a serious welfare problem and the veterinarian may be

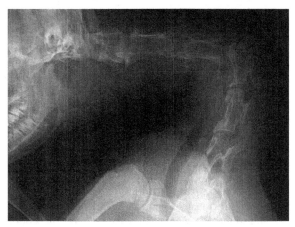

Fig. 6.20 – Deer. Immature roe deer caught by dogs. Neck dislocated by owner of dogs.

asked to provide a statement on the suffering involved. It is worth considering whether occlusion of the ear canals by inflammation and exudate may dull the hearing to the extent that the dog or cat is put at increased risk of being involved in a motor vehicle accident.

In farm livestock, fraudulent replacement of ear-tags often causes fresh holes in the ear-flap, and estimation of the time that has elapsed since the tag was changed can be crucial in these investigations. Microscopically, new holes show recent disruption of the cartilage and soft tissues. The margins are irregular and tattered, and show either no evidence of repair or only those changes related to early healing, e.g. partial epithelialisation and non-birefringent fibrous scarring. In contrast, long-standing ear-tag holes have rounded healed margins with the severed edges of the cartilage covered by mature scar tissue over which the skin has grown through the hole to complete the healing process. Chronic irritation in long-standing holes is characterised by a chronic inflammatory cell response and proliferation of scar tissue at the affected part of the hole margin.

Neck injuries

Dislocation and cervical fractures

Dislocation of the neck is a common method of killing birds and is used to dispatch farmed poultry, reared game birds and others. In a forensic context, such as illegal killing of protected species, radiographs are valuable to show the separation of the cervical vertebrae. At necropsy, the marked haemorrhage that accompanies rupture of blood vessels in the neck provides evidence that the bird was alive at the time of dislocation.

Dislocation of the cervical vertebrae is used as a method of immobilising or killing small deer that have been caught by hunting dogs. X-ray plates are invaluable in providing graphic evidence for the courts on this type of injury (Fig. 6.20).

Occasionally, attempts are made to kill kittens and dogs by 'breaking their necks'. This may be unsuccessful and the animal is then killed by some other means. Nevertheless, bruising in neck muscles and various degrees of haemorrhage within the spinal canal may provide corroborating evidence of the alleged initial attack.

Cervical fractures can occur in motor vehicle accidents and are accompanied by other evidence of such an accident. More concerning are explanations such as 'rough play' or 'falling in a hole'[10] and the veterinarian may wish to explore the circumstances carefully.

Ligature marks from strangulation

Externally there may be limited evidence of ligature marks in fatal strangulation because the hair and looseness of the skin around the neck can protect against skin abrasion. However, careful examination may reveal areas where there is indentation of hair or patchy loss of hair or reddening or mild bruising of the skin. Subcutaneous bruising may be present over the larynx, at the angle of the jaw or where the knot in the ligature has tightened against the neck. In badgers, there may be a linear subcutaneous mark indicating the line of the ligature (see Chapter 11: Traps and snares). It should be noted that the *absence* of ligature marks does not discount death by strangulation.

Chest injuries

Bruising

Bruising over the chest wall is a frequent and highly significant finding but reflection of the skin is absolutely necessary to appreciate the full extent of the bleeding. Blunt trauma is the major cause of chest wall bruising, although the position and nature of the haemorrhage may give little or no indication of its cause. Marked haemorrhage in the pectoral muscles can be associated with major blunt force trauma to the ventral or anterior parts of the chest wall. It may also develop following stab wounds or, in small creatures, bite injuries inflicted by large predators. Haemorrhage in large muscle groups can assume a streaky appearance when blood tracks along fascial planes. Forcible abduction of the forelegs in dogs can lead to tearing of blood vessels in the axillae with extensive and severe haemorrhage spreading over the chest wall.

The rib cages of young cats and dogs are extremely flexible and bend readily under blunt force trauma. When this happens, subcutaneous bruising may not develop (because the skin stretches and the subcutaneous blood vessels are not crushed against unyielding bone) but haemorrhage occurs in the intercostal muscles as these are torn during the distortion of the chest wall. Removal of the layer of fat overlying the ribs may be necessary to appreciate the distribution of this haemorrhage.

Haemorrhage over the dorsal third of the ribs may indicate compression or distortion of the chest with bending or fracture of ribs close to the spinal column (Fig. 6.21).

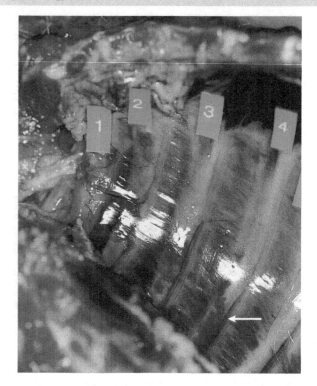

Fig. 6.21 – Adult dog. Punching and striking with a hammer resulted in multiple injuries to head and body of this terrier. Note haemorrhages over proximal ends of ribs 2, 3 and 4 (arrow) probably caused by bending of the ribs. Rib 3 was fractured close to the spine.

Rib fractures

Fractured ribs can be easily missed in X-rays taken during standard positioning for X-ray examination. Recent rib fractures are usually accompanied by haemorrhage, which is often easier to see on the pleural surface of the chest wall.

The pattern of rib fractures is not specific for particular events but should be viewed in the light of other injuries (or lack of them) and other circumstances of the case. Although uncommon in adequately nourished animals and birds, natural bone disease in the form of under-mineralisation should be considered in the differential diagnosis. Similarly, disseminated neoplasia may be a factor predisposing to rib fractures. The fact that natural disease is present does not, however, diminish culpability for neglect through lack of veterinary attention (see Chapter 5: Neglect, Case study 5.6). In flail chest with multiple rib fractures and consequent inability to inflate the lungs, death may supervene from asphyxia.

Lung, windpipe and heart injuries

Complications associated with fractured ribs include pneumothorax, haemothorax and puncturing of the lungs by the fractured rib ends. Substantial blunt trauma (motor vehicle accidents, falls from considerable heights or other heavy

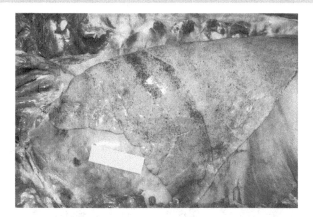

Fig. 6.22 – Pig. Fell from moving vehicle, sustaining multiple injuries including bruising in the lungs caused by the impact of the ribs.

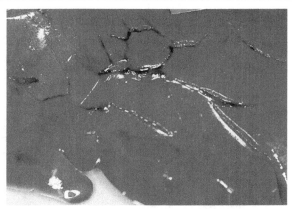

Fig. 6.23 – Puppy. Multiple ruptures of liver caused by forceful kicking of the abdomen led to fatal internal haemorrhage.

blows) to the chest may cause emphysematous bullae formation in the lung, laceration of lung lobes, bruising of the lungs with imprints of ribs (Fig. 6.22), or major haemorrhage arising from torn blood vessels in the soft tissues situated between the lungs (mediastinum).

In kittens, forcible stretching of the neck during attempted 'wringing or breaking of the neck' may lead to tracheal avulsion with the trachea becoming separated from the lung close to the bifurcation of the mainstem bronchi. The ante-mortem nature of the injury is confirmed by the demonstration of blood within the tracheal lumen and haemorrhage into the chest cavity.

Bruising of the heart may occur following severe blunt trauma to the chest but, in the authors' experience, appears to be uncommon. Similarly, rupture of the pericardium is rare.

Collection of a small volume of blood-stained fluid in the pericardial sac is a common finding after freezing and thawing of a body and should not be mistaken for ante-mortem intrapericardial haemorrhage.

Abdominal injuries

Bruising

It is important to note that lack of bruising to the abdominal wall does not correlate with an absence of serious injury to the abdominal organs. This is analogous to the situation in children where absence of abdominal bruising can lead to the assumption of no internal damage, with consequent diagnostic delay and high case fatality.[11]

Liver

Kicks and heavy blows can result in rupture of the liver. These ruptures may be single or multiple, and a pattern of 'crazing' is common (Fig. 6.23). The site of the blow, and the position of the animal at the time, both affect which lobe or lobes are damaged. Bleeding from a liver rupture is sometimes limited and characterised only by clots adhering to the surface around the split in the capsule. In contrast, multiple ruptures with major damage to the liver parenchyma can result in massive bleeding.

Spleen

Splenic injury appears less commonly than liver damage in dogs and cats that have been kicked or beaten. When it occurs, the spleen may be completely transected or show local capsular or subcapsular haemorrhage.

Kidneys

Blunt trauma may result in haemorrhage (retroperitoneal) around one or both kidneys, and blood-stained fluid in the urinary bladder may indicate renal damage that is not readily visible grossly. The kidneys may be extensively damaged in motor vehicle accidents if the body is crushed.

Dark post-mortem discoloration to the posterior pole of one or both kidneys is a common finding and is associated with bacterial activity in the loops of intestine that rest against the kidneys (Fig. 6.24). This colour change can be identified wrongly as bruising, and microscopic examination can aid in the differentiation where there is such doubt.

Stomach and intestines

Gross traumatic damage to hollow organs is uncommon in non-accidental injury. However, blunt trauma (e.g. kicks) can cause rupture of a distended stomach or result in intestinal perforation if a loop is impacted against the spinal column. Similar trauma may result in haemorrhage at the root of the mesentery with leakage down the mesentery towards the intestines.

Limb and pelvic injuries

Fractures of limb bones and the pelvis are common in companion animals and have a multitude of causes. All

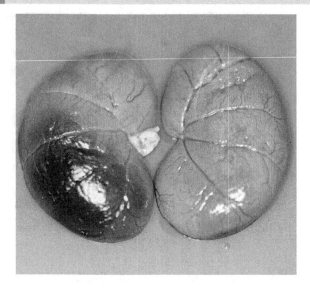

Fig. 6.24 – Cat. Post-mortem discoloration of kidney can be mistaken for bruising.

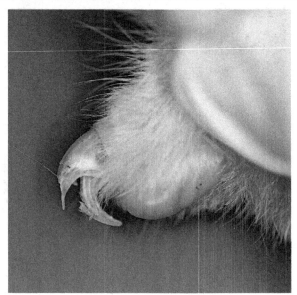

Fig. 6.26 – Cat. Broken claw in young cat that died from subdural haemorrhage caused by non-accidental head trauma.

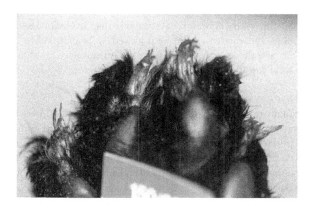

Fig. 6.25 – Cat. Tattered claws can provide supporting evidence of a motor vehicle accident or other struggle.

fractures should be assessed in the light of the history and the presence (or absence) of other injuries to the animal (see Chapter 3: Non-accidental injury).

Currently, there are no specific fractures, or combination of fractures, to limbs or pelvis that have been recognised as being caused exclusively by physical abuse. However, repeated fractures or fractures of different ages (in the absence of underlying bone pathology) raise concerns over the circumstances of the injuries.

Feet and claws

Tattering of the claws of cats that have been involved in motor vehicle accidents is well recognised by clinicians (Fig. 6.25). Similarly, arboreal animals that fall (e.g. pine martens) may tatter their claws as they try to slow their descent by grasping at lower branches. Breakage of claws

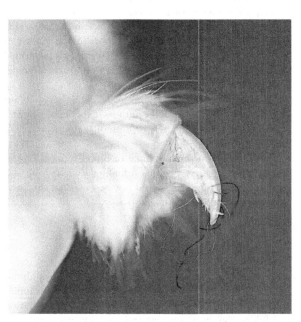

Fig. 6.27 – Cat. Fibres caught in claws may provide valuable samples in scenes of crime investigations.

may also occur when a cat makes strenuous attempts to escape any form of trauma (Fig. 6.26), and fibres caught in claws may be valuable to investigations by scene-of-crime officers, and should be retained (Fig. 6.27). Cats trapped in tumble dryers may cling strongly to the revolving drum, and suffer heat-related claw damage (Fig. 6.28).

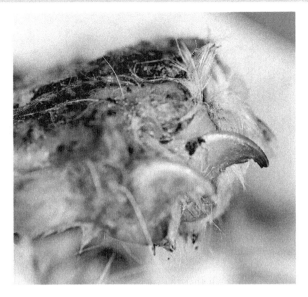

Fig. 6.28 – Cat. Killed in a tumble dryer. The claws of this cat showed heat discoloration at their tips.

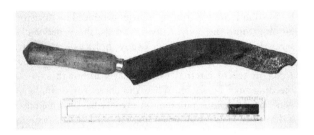

Fig. 6.29 – A 'turnip' knife. This was the type of weapon used to injure the cat shown in Fig. 6.30.

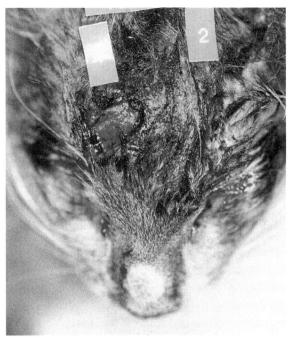

Fig. 6.30 – Cat. Incised wounds to the top of the head of a cat caused by blows from a relatively blunt knife.

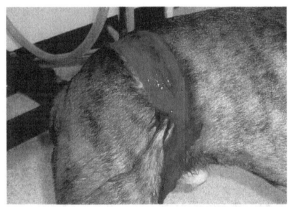

Fig. 6.31 – Staffordshire bull terrier. Slash wound caused by a sharp blade. Note profuse bleeding and sharp, cleanly cut, wound margins. (By kind permission of the Royal Society for the Prevention of Cruelty to Animals.)

Sharp force injuries

Incised wounds

Incised wounds are caused by sharp-edged objects (e.g. knives and broken glass) being drawn across the skin surface. They are often referred to as *cuts* or *slash wounds*.

Most non-accidental incised wounds in veterinary cases are inflicted by knives of varying types, including hunting knives and the blades of tools such as 'Stanley' or 'box' knives. Heavier weapons, such as 'samurai swords', bladed fighting sticks, machetes and pangas, are also used. Sometimes a relatively blunt blade (Fig. 6.29) may cause a wound that, on first examination, is not readily classified as 'incised' or 'lacerated' (Fig. 6.30). Such injuries are best described as 'cuts' until more is known about the type of weapon.

Incised wounds tend to be long relative to their depth, and have clean-cut edges devoid of abrasion or bruising. They bleed profusely (Fig. 6.31). The shape of an incised wound gives little indication of the nature or size of the cutting agent other than to confirm that it had a sharp edge (Fig. 6.32). Some incised wounds are deeper at the initial part of the cut and become shallower as the blade rises out of the wound at the opposite end. However, the interaction between the victim and the attacker is dynamic and no hard-and-fast rules apply to the shape or depth of the wound.

Incised wounds to the neck are inflicted during attempts to 'cut the throat'. These wounds may be found in the

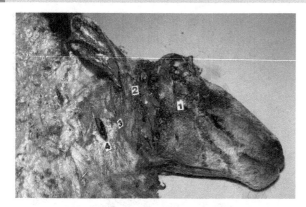

Fig. 6.32 – Sheep. Incised wounds in the skin caused by a relatively blunt 'Samurai' sword. Note that wound no. 1 has caused extensive damage to the bone at the margin of the eye socket, indicating a heavy blow.

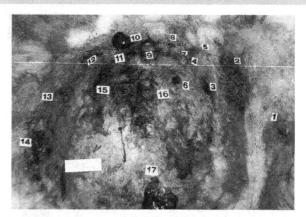

Fig. 6.35 – Sheep. Multiple stab wounds to the abdomen. Each stab wound is numbered for clarity.

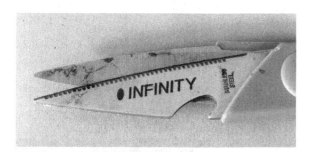

Fig. 6.33 – Scissors used to cut off the tip of the ear of an elderly dog during a prolonged sadistic attack culminating in the dog being bludgeoned to death with a hammer.

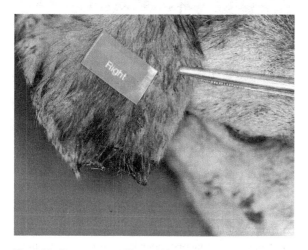

Fig. 6.34 – Same case as in Figure 6.33, showing cut end of ear.

middle to upper part of the neck on the ventral or lateral surfaces. Some cuts can be close to the angle of the jaw.

Sharp scissors can also cause incised wounds (Fig. 6.33). When scissors have been used to cut off the tip of an ear (Fig. 6.34) it may be difficult at post-mortem examination

to be certain whether the cut was inflicted by a knife or scissors.

Stab (puncture) wounds

Stab wounds are penetrating injuries produced by thrusting an object into the body. Knives, swords, sharpened sticks, screwdrivers, scissors and crossbow bolts are amongst a range of weapons that cause puncture wounds and may result in severe internal haemorrhage, although *external* bleeding may be *slight*. When the chest, for example, is penetrated, various pulmonary, myocardial and mediastinal injuries may result depending on the depth of penetration and the dynamics of the event. Pneumothorax, haemothorax, haemopericardium and cardiac tamponade are possible complications.

If there are multiple wounds, it is helpful if these are numbered before being photographed (Fig. 6.35).

The depth of a stab wound is usually considerably greater than the length of the skin wound. The exact shape of the penetrating object can rarely be deduced from the shape of skin wound. A double-edged knife blade *may* leave a skin wound that tapers at both ends, contrasting it with the hole made by a single-edged blade. However, an individual weapon may cause wounds of various shapes and sizes depending on the angle of attack, movement and tightness of the skin at the time and subsequently. *Consequently no reliance should be placed on the shape of a stab wound in the skin.* If the penetrating object is relatively blunt (e.g. a stick), the entry hole may show inversion of the margins where the skin was forced or dragged into the hole (Fig. 6.36).

The depth of a penetrating wound may give some indication of the length of the weapon, but not necessarily so. If the blade has not been inserted its full length, the wound will underestimate blade length. Conversely, a violent thrust may cause the knife to penetrate to the hilt and then to depress the abdominal wall, allowing the

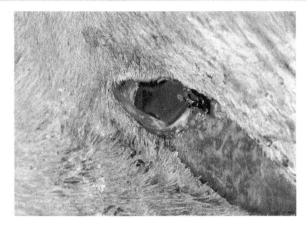

Fig. 6.36 – Horse. A penetrating wound by a pointed stick to the chest of a stallion punctured the heart. The slightly inverted upper margin of the wound indicates this is an entry wound rather than an exit hole.

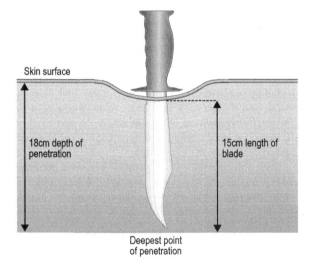

Skin surface

18cm depth of penetration

15cm length of blade

Deepest point of penetration

Fig. 6.37 – A forceful stab to the body may depress the wall allowing deeper organs to be injured, thereby creating a misleading impression of the blade length.

tip of the blade to penetrate deeper organs and thereby giving a misleading impression of the length of the blade (Fig. 6.37).

Perforating wounds are wounds that pass through the body, or part of the body, and result in an entry wound on one side and an exit wound on the other. They can be caused, for example, by stabs, bullets or arrows.

Angle of stab wound

The site of the injury (e.g. the side of the neck), angle of penetration and direction of a stab wound may provide clues to the posture adopted by the animal at the moment the injury occurred. For example, it may be claimed that stabbing was accidental, or carried out in self-defence, when a dog has (allegedly) leapt on a person carrying a

---

> ### Case study 6.6
>
> **Clinical history:**
> The owner (6 ft/1.83 metres tall) of a bullmastiff claimed that a fatal stab wound to the neck of the dog occurred when the dog leapt at him. He also stated that, at the time, he was holding a 'Chinese fighting stick' at approximately waist height. Shoulder height of the mastiff was approximately 26 inches (66 cm).
>
> **The issues:**
> The blade entered the left side of lower neck in front of the left shoulder, passing inwards towards midline and angled downwards to the front of the chest above the breastbone. The angle of this wound suggested that the dog was standing with his front feet on the ground. If this large dog had been rearing up on his hind legs, it is probable that the wound would have been *horizontal or angled upwards* (depending on the exact position of the dog at the time of impact of the blade) rather than being *angled downwards*.

knife. Reconstruction of the incident, however, using information on the height of the accused, the manner in which the weapon was held and the account of the incident may reveal inconsistencies that investigators may wish to explore (Case study 6.6).

Similarly the angle and direction of wounds inflicted by an assailant standing over an animal can be revealing. The stabbing action is generally downwards and inwards. If the assailant is right-handed and is astride a standing dog whilst lifting the chin to expose the underside of the neck, the wound will have a tendency to track from slightly to the right of midline towards the left side of the neck, slicing the trachea and severing the left jugular and carotid but sparing these vessels on the right side.

Force of stab wounds

The forces involved in stabbing attacks have been the focus of considerable research.[12-15] Much of this interest hinges on the crucial issue of whether the wounding was the result of an accident or an act of violence.

Although the object of the research was to seek answers relating to stabbing of people, some of the experiments were conducted on cadaveric pig material[13] and this is of direct interest to veterinarians. It is clear that:

* The sharpness of the point of the weapon has a great influence on the force required to puncture skin. The sharper the point, the less is the force needed. Tightly stretched skin is easier to puncture than slack, loose skin. Consequently, it may take less force to puncture the chest wall between the ribs than is required to penetrate the slack, relaxed abdominal wall.

* Data on the precise forces required to penetrate the skin of live companion animals are not available but the investigations on the biomechanics of knife stab

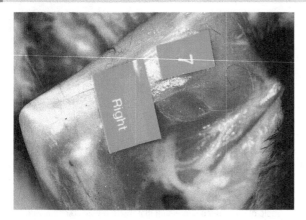

Fig. 6.38 – Cat. The injury to the muscle of the leg of this cat shows no evidence of bleeding and occurred after death. The wound in the overlying skin was similarly non-haemorrhagic. The cat died from other injuries caused by beating and stabbing.

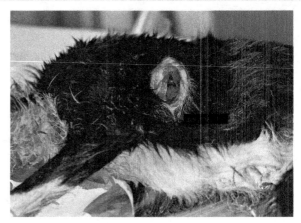

Fig. 6.39 – Dog. Mutilation of the chest after death. Note the lack of haemorrhage associated with this major wound to the chest.

attacks[15] indicate that very high-energy levels can be reached in overhand and side-swipe attacks, whereas thrusts tend to be lower in energy.

- It is also clear that the skin is the main barrier to penetrating wounds (other than striking bone or cartilage) and that the resistance of muscle to penetration is overcome by the follow-through action of stabbing. The resistance of muscle to penetration might, however, be of relevance when a projectile (e.g. a thrown knife) causes the stab wound and the initial impact with the skin ensures partial depletion of the projectile's kinetic energy.

Radiography may prove useful in demonstrating the extent of the force applied to an incised wound if underlying bones, such as cervical vertebrae, are damaged by the edge of the blade.

Post-mortem knife wounds

Cadavers are from time to time mutilated by stabbing or slashing. These injuries may be related to the cause of death in cases where the victim dies during the attack yet the stabbing or slashing continues (Fig. 6.38). Alternatively, the corpse of an animal (that has died from some unrelated cause) is subject to post-mortem mutilation (Fig. 6.39).

Dating of wounds

This is an area of forensic veterinary pathology that must be approached with considerable care. The reasons for this caution stem from the range of species that is involved and the complexity of the factors that may influence wound healing. Currently, to our knowledge, there are no robust data on the timing of the sequences of events that follow the progression of untreated, non-surgical wounds in domestic animals. The expected early reparative changes such as regrowth of damaged epithelium and formation of granulation tissue are well described in diagnostic pathology texts. However, the onset and development of these stages of repair are affected by a number of circumstances including infection, maggots, nutritional and immune states, and the animal's age. There is an urgent need for thorough investigation of the influences exerted by these factors on wound healing in different species of domestic and free-living animals and birds.

Some information on the ageing of bruises is presented earlier in this chapter. Other histopathological observations that may provide some guidance on wound healing are:

- 24 hours: serum/clot with congestion, swelling and leucocytic infiltration
- 36 hours: new capillaries
- 48–72 hours: spindle-shaped cells at right angles to the vessels
- 5–6 days: fibrils parallel to the vessels
- 21 days: birefringence developing in newly laid down bovine collagen.

The veterinarian may think that particular findings are simple and self-evident and, as a result, may fail to highlight their relevance. For example, it needs to be explained that the discovery of a shotgun pellet, wrapped in fibrous tissue and unaccompanied by haemorrhage, embedded in the side of the face of a spaniel is evidence of a shooting injury weeks, months or even years previously but is not related to shooting in the last few days. Similarly, the long-term nature of the wounds to the face of a bull caused by ingrowing horns (see Case study 5.5) would need to be spelled out.

With regard to fractures, proliferation of the periosteum (which gives rise to the external callus) may begin within

24 hours of injury. Early mineralisation of irregular trabeculae in the callus may be detectable by histopathological examination within 1 week, whereas radiographs may highlight mineralisation at around 2 weeks post-injury. Remodelling of the callus and removal of necrotic bone, however, can take many months or years depending on the bone, the type of injury, and the age and species of the animal.

References

1. Saukko P, Knight B. The pathology of wounds. In: Knight's forensic pathology, 3rd edn. London: Arnold; 2004:136–173.

2. McNally PW, Warris PD. Recent bruising in cattle at abattoirs. Vet Rec 1996; 138:126–128.

3. Bremner A, Johnston M, eds. Welfare of poultry at slaughter. In: Poultry meat hygiene and inspection. London: Saunders; 1996:53–72.

4. Gracey JF, Collins DS, Huey RJ. From farm to slaughter. In: Meat hygiene, 10th edn. London: Saunders; 1999: 163–196.

5. McCausland IP, Dougherty R. Histological ageing of bruises in lambs and calves. Aust Vet J 1978; 54:525–527.

6. Kleinman PK, Barnes PD. Head trauma. In: Kleinman PK, ed. Diagnostic imaging of child abuse, 2nd edn. Mosby, 1998:285–342.

7. Saukko P, Knight B. Head and spinal injuries. In: Knight's forensic pathology, 3rd edn. London: Arnold; 2004:174–221.

8. Munro HMC, Thrusfield MV. 'Battered pets': non-accidental physical injuries found in dogs and cats. J Small Anim Pract 2001; 42:279–290.

9. Barnett KC, Crispin SM, eds. Fundus. In: Feline ophthalmology. Edinburgh: Elsevier Science; 2002:146–183.

10. Hawthorne JC, Blevins WE, Wallace LJ et al. Cervical vertebral fractures in 56 dogs: a retrospective study. J Am Hosp Assoc 1999; 35:135–146.

11. Hobbs CJ, Hanks HG, Wynne JM. Physical abuse. In: Child abuse and neglect. A clinician's handbook, 2nd edn. London: Churchill Livingstone; 1999:63–104.

12. Knight B. The dynamics of stab wounds. Forensic Sci 1975; 6:249–255.

13. Jones S, Nokes L, Leadbeatter S. The mechanics of stab wounding. Forensic Sci Int 1994; 67:59–63.

14. O'Callaghan PT, Jones MD, James DS et al. Dynamics of stab wounds: force required for penetration of various cadaveric human tissues. Forensic Sci Int 1999; 104:173–178.

15. Chadwick EKJ, Nicol AC, Lane JV et al. Biomechanics of knife attacks. Forensic Sci Int 1999; 105:35–44.

7 | Thermal Injuries

Introduction

Thermal injuries are caused by:

- Direct (contact) heat such as a flame, hot surface (including electrocution burns) or hot liquid
- Radiant heat, e.g. a dog lying close to but not touching a wood burning stove
- Microwave radiation in a microwave oven
- Hyperthermia related to excessive ambient temperature (see Chapter 10)
- Hypothermia and frostbite (see Chapter 10).

Direct and radiant heat injuries tend to be localised, whereas the lesions of hyperthermia and hypothermia may be more generalised.

Prime questions for the forensic practitioner are:

- What caused the injury?
- When did it happen?
- Was it an accident?
- What are the differential diagnoses?

Many thermal injury studies have been conducted on experimental animals. Most of these experiments are focused on specific aspects of immunosuppression, chemicals released, or translocation of bacteria in animals burned experimentally. Readers wishing to delve more deeply into the detail of the cellular and systemic reactions of thermal injury should consider the ethics of using data generated by such experiments and the potential dangers of interpretation when laboratory results from one species are relied upon in the context of a forensic examination of a different species.

Burns

As a general principle, it is useful to remember that burns are often distributed asymmetrically or are localised, whereas a condition such toxic epidermal necrolysis has a symmetrical pattern and wide distribution. The shape of lesions may also be helpful in deciding on whether the lesions are burns. According to Gross et al (p 96)[1] '*Biologically abnormal patterns such as straight or angular borders, drip configurations or unusual symmetry*' may increase the index of suspicion of a burn.

Burns tend not to progress after about 5 days (unless there is repetitive injury) and this may be a useful feature in the differentiation from other skin lesions. The differen-

tial diagnosis of these types of lesion is addressed in standard dermatology texts.[1,2]

Traditionally, burns to domestic animals are divided into three categories.[1]

Superficial: first degree

Cellular damage is confined to the epidermis, although a vascular reaction in the dermis results in erythema and oedema.

Partial thickness: second degree

Coagulative epidermal necrosis is accompanied by hypereosinophilic epithelial cells, shrunken or karyorrhectic nuclei, dermal oedema and spongiosis. Vesicles and bullae form in the epidermis often at the epidermal–dermal junction. The bullae contain serum, glandular debris and leukocytes.

Full thickness: third degree

As the name suggests, the injury involves the full thickness of the skin. Coagulative necrosis develops in the connective tissue, blood vessels and skin adnexae. Microscopically, the epidermis and dermis may have a swollen amorphous appearance before neutrophilic inflammation becomes established. Granulomatous panniculitis is more suggestive of thermal injury than chemical burns (see Chapter 10).

Burns caused by flame

Flames singe hair and feathers before more serious damage (charring) develops in the skin, nails, beaks and deeper tissues. Careful examination of the pattern of hair or feather damage can help establish the position adopted by the victim at the time of being burnt or engulfed in flame (Case studies 7.1–7.3, Figs 7.1–7.6).

Dogs that survive burning may show scarring and loss of hair at various sites together with deformities of ear-flaps and foot-pads (Case study 7.4, Fig. 7.7).

Examination of burnt cadaver

It is unusual for the forensic veterinary pathologist to attend the scene where the body is found. During handling and transportation to the laboratory some changes are almost

Case study 7.1

A nest of baby birds in a hedgerow was doused with inflammable liquid and set alight during a domestic dispute. Four chicks that were partially decomposed and infested by maggots were submitted for examination. All chicks had been eating shortly before death and no life-threatening natural disease could be recognised at necropsy.

Charring affected feathers, beaks, wing tips, hocks and feet, and in one chick the sternum was burnt. Particles of burnt material were present on the body surfaces and, in one chick, deep within the air passages of the lungs. Some parts of the surface of each chick were unaffected. Using this pattern of exposed, burned areas and unburned parts (which were protected either by the wall of the nest or as a result of being pressed tightly against siblings), it was possible to reconstruct the situation in the nest at the time of the fire. A simple diagrammatic representation of the nest and chicks allowed the Court to visualise and understand why certain parts were burned and others spared (Fig. 7.1).

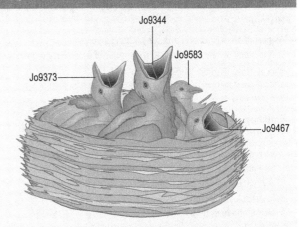

Fig. 7.1 – A hand-drawn illustration included in a veterinary report can be helpful to the Court. In this case, the pattern of burning on the various birds allowed reconstruction of their position in the nest.

Case study 7.2

A report was received of two men dousing a young pigeon in cigarette lighter fuel, or similar inflammable liquid, before setting the bird on fire. When questioned, the accused admitted setting the bird alight but claimed that the bird was dead, lying on her back. Burnt feathers showed that flames had extended over the back from the tail, the head, and along the under surface around the vent and posterior abdomen (but not the breast), and undersurface of the right wing. Extending the left wing (Fig. 7.2) revealed that the feathers at the wing tip, and over part of the back of the bird, were undamaged. These areas of burning indicate that the pigeon was resting on her chest with her right wing extended but the left wing held tightly against the body.

The marked hyperaemia of the right side of the head (Fig. 7.3) and of the left foot (Fig. 7.2) is a vital reaction and confirms that the bird survived the attack for a limited period. Internally there was no evidence of natural disease or other trauma that might account for disability or death of this bird.

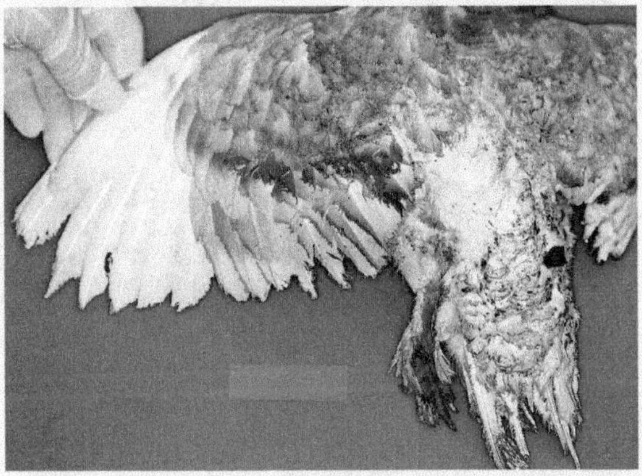

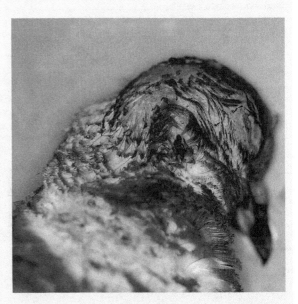

Fig. 7.2 – Pigeon. The pattern of singeing of feathers indicates the posture adopted at the time of burning.

Fig. 7.3 – Pigeon. The hyperaemia (visible on head) is a vital reaction that indicates that the bird was alive at the time of burning.

Case study 7.3

History:

As part of an intimidation attack by a gang involved in serious crime, a bull terrier belonging to a member of a competing gang was seized. He was secured to a railing by his chain collar, cut and stabbed with a knife, and then burned to death on a fire set beneath him.

Findings:

1. The skin over most of the body had a parchment-like texture with the most advanced charring affecting the head, shoulders and anterior chest. The subcutaneous muscles of the head and shoulders had a fawn, partially cooked, appearance. The impression of the chain was deeply embedded in the burnt skin of the neck (Fig. 7.4).

2. Extensive laceration and splitting of skin had occurred over the anterior chest, left shoulder (Fig. 7.5) and anterior surface of the left foreleg between elbow and metacarpus.

3. The frontal bone and the left zygomatic arch were fractured. Considerable quantities of blood had collected in the frontal sinuses. There was fragmentation and loss of teeth in the left upper jaw.

4. Findings in the respiratory tract included pooling of blood in the larynx and upper windpipe, blood-stained froth in the upper windpipe, moderate quantities of blood and mucus in the lower windpipe and main bronchi, marked congestion and flooding of the lungs together with numerous inhaled carbon particles in the air sacs of the lungs (Fig. 7.6).

Interpretation:

The blood in the frontal sinuses suggested that the skull fractures had occurred before death.

The blood, froth and carbon particles through the respiratory tract clearly indicated that the dog was alive whilst in the fire.

The splitting of the skin in burnt cadavers must be viewed with some caution. Splits are known to arise in the heated skin of burnt human corpses,[3] particularly over extensor surfaces and joints; the same may be true for domestic animals. Such splits can mimic ante-mortem wounds and need to be differentiated from true wounds. This may be difficult if heat damage is considerable, but examination of deeper tissues may provide convincing evidence of ante-mortem wounding.

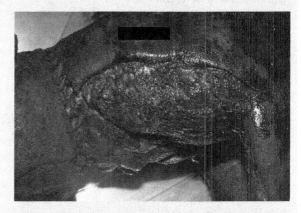

Fig. 7.5 – Same case as in Figure 7.4. A large split in the skin is present over the left shoulder. Care needs to be taken to differentiate splits in heated skin from ante-mortem injuries.

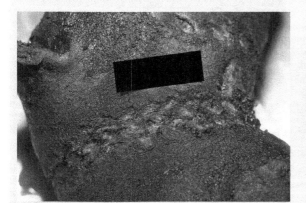

Fig. 7.4 – Staffordshire bull terrier. The burnt skin retained a deep impression of the chain around his neck.

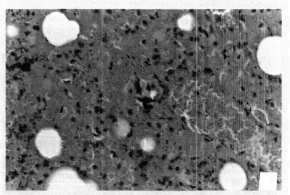

Fig. 7.6 – Same case as in Figure 7.4. Numerous inhaled carbon particles are visible in this congested, flooded lung.

Case study 7.4

Milly's owner left her in his apartment, which he had deliberately set on fire. She suffered severe burns to her head (ears, nose and around both eyes) and the pads of all four feet (Fig. 7.7).

After being rescued by a large (and angry) fire officer, she was adopted by a new family who gave her all the care she needed. Her burns gradually healed and she slowly recovered, although her face and ears were permanently scarred. Her feet seemed to be tender in cold weather, and she sometimes needed to wear boots to protect them.

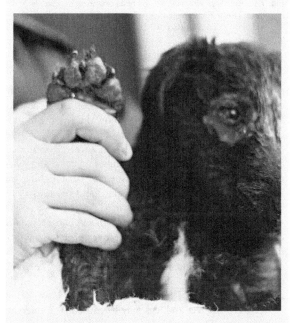

Fig. 7.7 – Milly. Note burns around eye and on pads of right forefoot. (By kind permission of the Scottish Society for the Prevention of Cruelty to Animals.)

Protocol A

- Incise under the chin and jaw, release the tongue and inspect the pharynx. Particles adhering to the mucous membranes of the pharynx and epiglottis may be scraped off with a clean scalpel blade and stored in a suitable glass bottle. Discard the blade.
- Inspect and photograph the glottis before inserting a gauze plug.
- In mammals, remove the entire respiratory tract together with the heart and set carefully to one side. Any deposits of burnt material that have flaked from the body should be collected or carefully covered by cloths to prevent soiling of the organs.
- In birds, open the ribcage and shine a bright white light on the airsacs to highlight inhaled particles.
- *Before* proceeding with further dissection, change gloves, apron and instruments.
- Note gross appearance of the lungs.
- Open the trachea through the dorsal membranous wall (paries membranacea) immediately posterior to the larynx and inspect the interior of the upper part of the windpipe, under a bright white light, for particles of burnt material. Shine the light forward into the posterior larynx and check for particulate matter on the mucous membrane. (The laryngeal wall can be relatively hard in older animals and, to avoid possible contamination further down the tract as the larynx is cut, it is better to leave further dissection of the larynx until the remainder of respiratory tract has been inspected and sampled.)
- Open the windpipe to the bifurcation and examine the mainstem bronchi. (Fresh gloves and instruments should be used to open the bronchi.)
- Collect samples of all lobes into 10% formalin for microscopic examination.
- Open the larynx.
- Examine mucus or froth samples under a dissecting microscope.

inevitable and the pathologist should make every effort to minimise any further loss of evidence or development of artefacts. It is important that the respiratory tract is secured against accidental contamination by burnt material. Protocol A gives confidence that any foreign matter found in the airways was not introduced by the pathologist.

Cigarette burns

Although the infliction of cigarette burns on abused companion animals is widely acknowledged to occur, there are no published descriptions of confirmed lesions. In children, cigarette burns are recognised by their size and shape (5–10 mm in diameter, circular and often of full thickness, creating a depressed crater[4]). In companion animals, one or more roughly circular, non-progressive lesions (on the head, forehead, face and dorsal surfaces of the forelegs or paws), possibly of different ages and of variable depth, may raise suspicions of deliberate burning by cigarettes (see Case study 5.6 & Fig. 7.8).

Other contact burns

Two factors are of particular relevance in the causation of contact burns: the length of time in contact with the hot surface and the temperature of the hot surface. Higher temperatures may instantly result in serious burns. In pigs, for

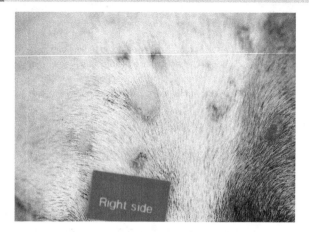

Fig. 7.8 – Staffordshire bull terrier. Suspected healing cigarette burns of different ages on forehead.

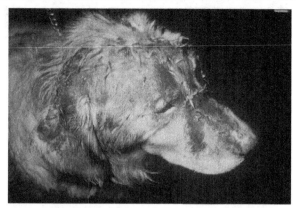

Fig. 7.9 – Retriever. Hot oil scalds on head extending to right ear and on to face. These were non-accidental injuries inflicted by the owner. (By kind permission of the Scottish Society for the Prevention of Cruelty to Animals.)

example, less than 1 second of contact at 70°C is sufficient to cause 'transepidermal' necrosis.[5]

Heated pads

The heated pads used in veterinary surgeries to protect debilitated patients (and those undergoing surgery or recovering from anaesthesia) from hypothermia may cause burns if they are in contact with the skin for extended periods.[6] A number of factors that influence the likelihood of burning include: nature of animal coat, insulation between pad and patient, and weight of patient. If burns occur there is a possibility of litigation, so records of pad temperature, duration of time on the pad and frequency of monitoring of patient could be important.

Hot iron disbudding

Thermal disbudding of goats can be a hazardous procedure because of the comparative thinness of goat kid skull. Heat from the disbudding iron may result in necrosis extending through the skin and frontal bones into the frontal cortex. The brain injury may range from polio-encephalomalacia to necrosis with cavitation, secondary infection and suppurative meningoencephalitis.[7]

Electrocution and lightning strike

Burns associated with suspected electrocution and lightning strike are considered in Chapter 10: Injuries associated with physical agents.

Scalds

Scalds are caused by contact with hot liquids, e.g. water and cooking oil. The contact occurs through splashing, pouring or immersion. When hot fluid has poured on to the skin, the lesions are frequently over the top of the head or face or back, and the pattern may show the flowing motion of the liquid. The full depth of the skin may be involved, but this can vary from lesion to lesion in the same animal. Scalds may be neglected over a number of days, and when presented for examination the tissue may be sloughing and infected. Healed scalds may be scarred and hairless.

The distribution of the scalds may direct the veterinarian to question the history offered to explain them. For example, a pan of boiling water overturned by a dog jumping up to the stove might well result in scalds to the chest and forelegs, but such a history would be an unlikely explanation for scalds in the middle of the back or on the top of the head (Fig. 7.9).

Scalds to the feet and legs may be caused by immersion in hot water. The depth of water is a crucial factor, with shallow water resulting in localised damage to pads and on to the upper surface of the digits. On contact with hot liquid cats contract the toes, which effectively protects the areas between the pads from the heat. Consequently, the pattern of injury to the foot in these shallow water cases consists of:

- loss of epithelium from the ventral surfaces of the pads with weeping or darkening of these lesions (depending on the time that has elapsed since the incident) (Fig. 7.10)
- normally coloured, non-erythematous areas between the pads and between the toes. The hairs on the ventral surface of the foot show no evidence of singeing (Fig. 7.10)
- reddening of the skin with loss of hair and epidermis on the lateral and dorsal aspects of the toes or foot, if splashing has occurred or if the water was sufficiently deep (Fig. 7.11).

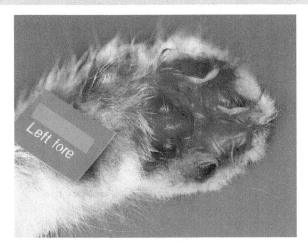

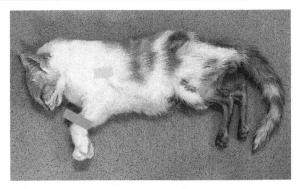

Fig. 7.12 – Cat. Forcible immersion of the hind limbs into hot water caused extensive deep scalding.

Fig. 7.10 – Kitten. Accidental scalding of feet in shallow water. Note detachment of the epidermis of digit pads 2, 3 and 4, reddening of the central part of the metacarpal pad, darkening of digit pad 5 and absence of singed hairs.

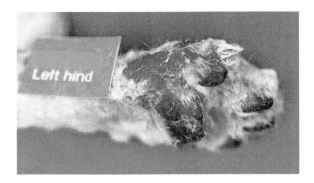

Fig. 7.11 – Same case as in Figure 7.10. Splashing of water has caused scalding over the side and on to the top surface of this foot.

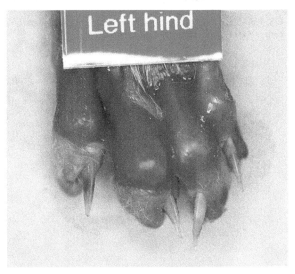

Fig. 7.13 – Same case as in Figure 7.12. Note apparent sparing of the skin at the distal ends of the toes.

Where one or more legs have been forcibly immersed in hot liquid, the lesions may extend some distance up the legs. There may be loss of hair and darkening and necrosis of the skin (Fig. 7.12). The upper margin of the scald may form a clearly defined line reminiscent of the so-called 'stocking' or 'glove' distribution in a child whose leg or hand has been deliberately immersed in hot water. A curious feature that is sometimes encountered in foot scalds in cats is the relative sparing of the skin immediately proximal to the nail beds (Fig. 7.13).

Microwave

Microwaves are electromagnetic waves in the range 1000–300 000 MHz. Microwave ovens pass microwave radiation, usually at a frequency of 2450 MHz, through food. Water, fat, sugar and certain other molecules absorb energy from the microwave beam and the vibration of the molecules creates heat.[8] Because the surrounding air does not warm up there is a common misconception that microwaves 'cook from the inside out'. Actually, it is the tissue with the highest water content that first heats up. Short exposure to microwaves may fail to cause obvious macroscopic damage to skin and organs. However, extended times in the oven result in cooking of the cadaver and its internal organs.

There is a paucity of published accounts of cases where small companion animals have been either killed or burned in microwave ovens. A toy poodle[9] was reported to have suffered multiple burns, midline on the dorsal thorax, after only 30 seconds' exposure to microwaves, but these injuries appear much too severe to have been caused by such brief exposure.

In the authors' experience, the spectrum of changes seen in cats placed in microwave ovens is wide and is almost certainly influenced by the duration of exposure and the power of the oven. In fatal cases, the features that raise suspicion of microwave damage are:

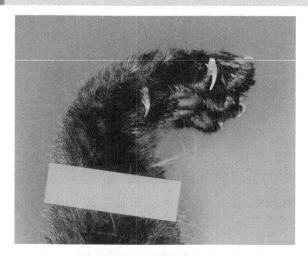

Fig. 7.14 – Cat, killed in a microwave oven. Flexure of the forefoot at the carpus and ex-sheathing of the claws are visible.

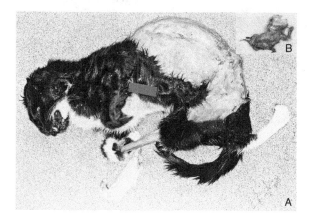

Fig. 7.15 – This pregnant cat was struck on the head and placed in a microwave oven for an extended period. She showed marked fragility of the skin and generally had a 'cooked' appearance. Her fetuses (inset) also had a cooked appearance.

- Flexure of the forelimb at the carpus with or without ex-sheathing of the claws (Fig. 7.14)
- Fragility of the skin that can lead to extensive splitting (with sharp, well delineated, edges) and slackening of the hair (Fig. 7.15)
- Absence of burning or singeing of hair
- Possible crumpling and reddening of the tips of the ear-flaps
- Congestion of all lobes of the lung with or without microscopic evidence of alveolar flooding and perivascular haemorrhage
- Internal organs may have a cooked appearance depending on the length of time in the oven. These cadavers may have a 'cooked chicken' odour and the tissues disintegrate readily.

References

1. Gross LE, Ihrke PJ, Walder EJ, Affolter VK, eds. Skin diseases of the dog and cat. Clinical and histopathologic diagnosis, 2nd edn. Oxford: Blackwell Science; 2005.
2. Scott DW, Miller WH, Griffin CE. Burns. In: Muller and Kirk's small animal dermatology, 6th edn. Philadelphia: Saunders; 2001:1083–1089.
3. Saukko P, Knight B. Burns and scalds. In: Knight's forensic pathology, 3rd edn. London: Arnold; 2004:312–325.
4. Hobbs CJ, Wynne JM. Other burn injuries. In: Physical signs of child abuse. London: W B Saunders; 2001:159–174.
5. Moritz AR, Henriques FC. Studies of thermal injury. II: The relative importance of time and surface temperature in the causation of cutaneous burns. Am J Pathol 1947; 23:695–720.
6. Swain SF, Lee AH, Hughes KS. Heating pads and thermal burns in small animals. J Am Anim Hosp Assoc 1989; 25:156–162.
7. Thompson KG, Bateman RS, Morris PJ. Cerebral infarction and meningoencephalitis following hot-iron disbudding of goat kids. N Z Vet J 2005; 53:368–370.
8. Encyclopaedia Britannica. Microwave oven. Online. Available: http://www.britannica.com/eb/article 5 Jun 2007.
9. Reedy LM, Clubb FJ. Microwave burn in a toy poodle: a case report. J Am Anim Hosp Assoc 1991; 27:497–500.

8 | Firearms Injuries

Introduction

Every year, millions of animals are shot. Most of this shooting is sanctioned by society and is not illegal. Veterinarians may, however, become involved in cases where the gunshot injury is:

- accidental
- involves damage to or destruction of property
- the public was endangered at the time the animal was shot
- the shooting was illegal because of the following:
  (a) restrictions relating to permissions to shoot
  (b) closed seasons for shooting
  (c) statutory protection of specified species of birds or mammals
  (d) the shooting caused unnecessary suffering to the animals.

If the veterinarian is to contribute meaningfully to any investigation involving firearms, it is necessary to have a basic understanding of the types of weapon used and the characteristics of the injuries caused by the various projectiles.

Air-rifles, shotguns and rifles cause the most common firearms injuries encountered by veterinarians in domestic and free-living animals. Handgun injuries do occur but are less frequent.

Types of weapon

Air-powered weapons

These range from simple, low-powered, smooth-bored guns, usually referred to as 'air-guns', to sophisticated high-powered air-rifles. The power is delivered by air that is compressed by the action of cocking the weapon or by pumping a lever. In gas-powered weapons, compressed carbon dioxide from a disposable cylinder is used. Air-powered weapons fire single pellets. The common calibres for air-powered weapons are 0.177, 0.2, 0.22 and 0.25 inches.

Shotgun

These weapons are single or double barrelled. The barrels are smooth-bored and the shotgun discharges multiple pellets in a mass each time it is fired. There is a variety of barrel lengths and calibres,[1] the calibre of the barrel usually being referred to as the 'bore' or 'gauge'. The 12-bore (0.729 inches/18.2 mm) is probably the most commonly used shotgun. An exception to the classification of 'bore' size is the '410', which refers to the actual diameter of the barrel (0.410 inches) and is the smallest of the commonly encountered shotguns.

Rifles

Rifles are characterised by having spiral grooves along the length of the internal surface of the barrel. These grooves cause the bullet to rotate along its longitudinal axis and this rotation, or spin, stabilises the bullet and prevents it from turning end over end whilst it is travelling through the air.

There are many calibres of rifle. Common hunting rifle calibres include .22, .243 and .270 (range 5.7–7 mm).[2] Rifles are further categorised by the method of ignition of the explosive charge in the cartridge. Those in which the firing pin strikes the rim of the cartridge are known as 'rimfire', whereas those that strike a central primer in the cartridge are called 'centrefire' rifles.

Generally, rimfire rifles are restricted to the ubiquitous .22 calibre, firing solid-nosed or hollow-nosed bullets with muzzle velocities ranging from 1000 to 1500 feet per second (fps). Centrefire rifles fire bullets with considerably greater muzzle velocities: 2400–4000 fps.

Ammunition

Air-rifle pellets

The pellets used in air-guns and air-rifles are the same, and are usually constructed of soft lead. The diabolo type of pellet has a narrow waist and a rounded point. Other lead pellets have straight sides and a more conical point. In the 'Prometheus', a polished zinc head is enveloped in a flexible synthetic jacket. This pellet is reputed to be capable of penetrating steel and so may be potentially more dangerous in head injuries.[3] The 'Sabo' pellet is also of compound construction, having lead and plastic components. Fragmentation of these two types of pellet can result in separation of the radio-opaque head of the pellet from the radio-lucent nylon or plastic part that remains within the wound track.

'BB' ammunition for air-guns is spherical lead shot that derives its name from the original method of describing the

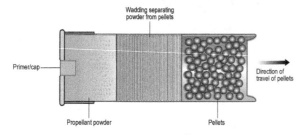

Fig. 8.1 – Diagrammatic representation of the main elements of a shotgun cartridge.

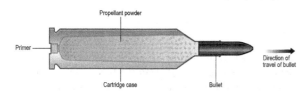

Fig. 8.2 – Diagrammatic representation of the main elements of a rifle bullet.

size of the lead balls. In this case, the shot size was between 'B' and 'BBB'.

Shotgun cartridges

The cartridge (Fig. 8.1) consists of several parts:

- The cartridge case (made of plastic or paper), with its steel head and primer, surrounds and contains the other components.
- The explosive charge known as 'powder'.
- Wadding, which separates the powder from the shotgun pellets.
- Shotgun pellets (there may be more than 200 pellets, depending on the size of the individual pellets) that are, most commonly, made of lead but some are steel, bismuth or tungsten, or copper-coated lead.

Rifle bullets

The cartridge case is usually of copper/zinc and contains the primer at the flat end and the propellant (explosive charge) in the middle part. At the forward end, the cartridge case is crimped around the bullet that protrudes from the point (Fig. 8.2).

The bullet can be solid in construction (usually lead) and may be covered by a very thin layer of copper. Lead bullets

are suitable only for rimfire weapons. Centrefire ammunition has a lead or steel core covered by a metal jacket that prevents the bullet melting or fragmenting as it travels down the barrel at high velocity. Most hunting ammunition has a 'partial metal jacket', meaning that the tip of the bullet is non-jacketed in order to maximise deformation of the bullet when striking the target.

Examination of a suspected firearms injury case

If possible, the whole bird or animal should be placed in a suitable bag, although clearly this may be impractical for large animals. Having the specimen properly bagged overcomes the problem of losing shotgun pellets or fragments of bullet that are lying on the surface of the skin or in the hair or feathers. Additionally, bagging will reduce the likelihood of 'cross-contamination' between specimens during storage or transportation.

Radiography

After initial examination of the outside of the body for evidence of bleeding or matted hair and feathers, a series of radiographs of the head, body and limbs, including the feet, may provide the first tangible evidence of pellets or bullet fragments.

Radiographs are of great assistance in the search for pellets or bullet fragments at post-mortem examination. However, to overcome the limitations inherent in the two-dimensional nature of radiographs, it is essential to have dorsoventral and lateral views. In addition, radiographs may indicate the track of the bullet through the body. This is of particular importance if the bullet has exited from the body.

Radiographs can aid in establishing, early in the investigation, which type of weapon was used (shotgun, rifle or air-rifle). Fragmentation patterns, as seen in radiographs, can be helpful in identifying the type of ammunition. For example, on striking dense bone, low-velocity .22 bullets break into a variable number of large and small radio-opaque fragments (Fig. 8.3). The greater energy associated with high-velocity bullets causes these bullets to disintegrate to a greater extent and may result in the fragmentation pattern commonly known as a 'lead snowstorm' (Fig. 8.4).

Separation of the core of a hunting bullet from the copper jacket may result in exit of the core with retention of the jacket in the cadaver. Rifling marks, used by ballistics experts to match bullets to suspect rifles, are present on the jackets of jacketed bullets and radiographic examination will assist in recovery of these valuable fragments.

On rare occasions, very forcible fracture of, for example, the femur of a fit and energetic horse can result in wounds caused by exiting bone fragments. These may be mistaken for bullet wounds. Radiography provides reassurance that firearms were not involved.

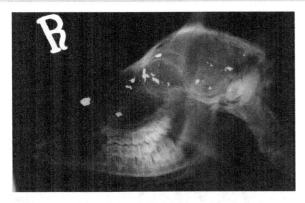

Fig. 8.3 – Radiograph of roe deer head showing the fragmentation pattern of a low-velocity .22 bullet extending from the back of the head to the nose.

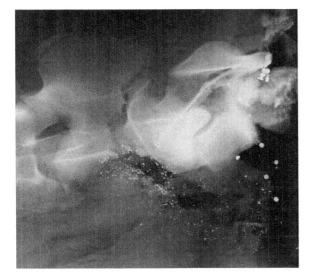

Fig. 8.4 – Radiograph of bull's neck showing fragmentation pattern ('lead snowstorm') of a fragile, high-velocity bullet (.22–.250) commencing at the skin and extending to the spinal column. Note also a small number of shotgun pellets at the right side.

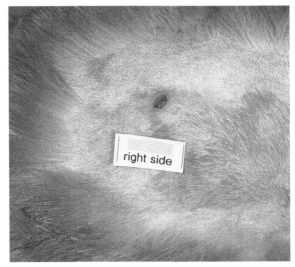

Fig. 8.5 – Cat showing entrance hole of a .22 bullet in the right flank. This hole was visible only after hair clipping.

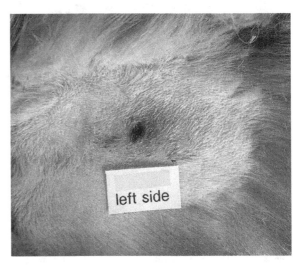

Fig. 8.6 – Cat (as in Fig. 8.5) showing exit hole in left side. This hole is marginally larger than the entrance hole and shows a halo of bruising.

Firearm wounds

General

In most cases the entry holes, and to a lesser extent the exit holes, will be obscured by hair or feathers. Clipping the hair or careful plucking of the feathers is necessary to reveal the skin wounds (Figs 8.5 & 8.6). Clipping the entire side of an animal will give a clear indication of the scatter of shotgun pellet injury (Fig. 8.7). Depending on the stance, position or action of the victim (e.g. flying, running, stretching, jumping), the skin wounds may or may not lie directly over deeper injuries found at post-mortem examination. Initial observations should include a description of surrounding bruising and the size and shape of hole. Fre-

quently, feathers or tufts of hair are drawn into an entry hole and provide convincing evidence that penetration occurred at these sites. Usually these hairs or feathers are found in the skin or subcutaneous tissues, but on occasion they may penetrate more deeply to the body cavities and the internal organs (Fig. 8.8).

Care needs to be exercised with the interpretation of exit wounds because fragments of bone rather than bullet may cause these, or because only part of the bullet may have exited.

The damage caused by pellets or bullets is related to the amount of kinetic energy possessed by the pellets or bullets and how much of this energy is transferred from the pellet

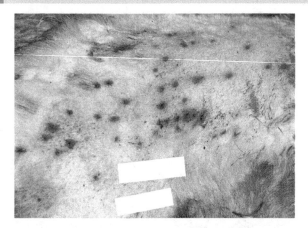

Fig. 8.7 – Clipped side of 7-month-old Labrador dog with widespread shotgun pellet entry holes following a 'distant' shot.

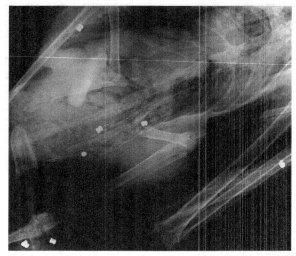

Fig. 8.9 – Radiograph of an adult swan shot seven times with air-rifle pellets.

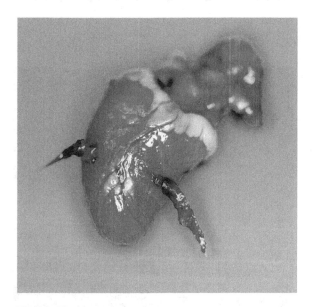

Fig. 8.8 – Feather drawn into and through the heart of a barn owl by a shotgun pellet.

or bullet to the tissues of the animal. The formula used to calculate kinetic energy is $E = (\frac{1}{2}) mv^2$, where E is the kinetic energy, m is the mass and v the velocity. Small, low-speed projectiles possess limited energy and therefore may cause limited tissue damage. Heavy, high-speed bullets have abundant kinetic energy and the potential to cause massive tissue injury.

Air-powered weapon wounds

Pellets fired from air-rifles are light in weight, travel at relatively low speeds and, consequently, have limited kinetic energy. In small mammals and birds the available energy is sufficient to cause fatal injury, but in larger creatures air-

rifle pellets frequently cause injuries that are not immediately fatal. In these cases it is common to find several pellets in one cadaver as a result of repeated attempts to kill the unfortunate animal (Fig. 8.9). However, exceptions do occur where a pellet causes rapid death following rupture of a major blood vessel or damage to a vital centre in the brain.

Entry holes are small (3–5 mm in diameter) and round or oval in shape. Bruising may develop around the margin of the hole. Perforating wounds, in which the pellet passes through the body or limb, entering one surface and exiting on the opposite side, can occur in small birds and mammals. The exit hole in these cases may be somewhat larger that the entry hole and are frequently elliptical because of distortion of the pellet or because of the angle of the pellet as it exits.

The track of the pellet in soft tissues is narrow and generally haemorrhagic. Abdominal wounds may result in rupture of several loops of intestines, release of intestinal contents and death from peritonitis some days after the shooting. Injuries to eyes are common in a range of domestic animals from cats to horses, and in wildlife from seals to raptors. Damage to the eye is often devastating.

One or more pellets related to previous shooting injuries may be found after a second fatal attack. On radiography the original pellets are not readily distinguishable from the more recent ones. However, at necropsy the older pellets are found to be partially or completely encapsulated in fibrous tissue and recent haemorrhage is not associated with their presence.

Shotgun wounds

The character of a shotgun wound is highly dependent on the discharge distance of the shot. At close range the

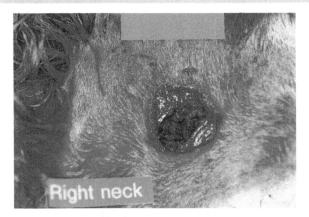

Fig. 8.10 – Neck wound in Labrador (as in Fig. 8.7) caused by discharge of a 12-bore shotgun at a distance of approximately 4 feet.

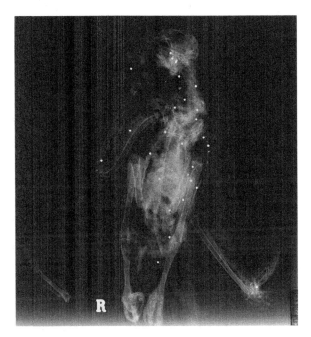

Fig. 8.11 – Radiograph of buzzard fatally wounded by a 'distant' shotgun. Note spread of pellets from head to tail and both wings.

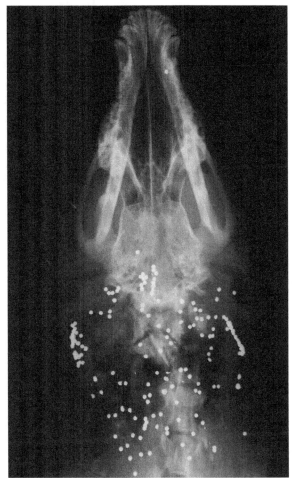

Fig. 8.12 – Radiograph showing clustering of shotgun pellets in Labrador's neck (see Fig. 8.10).

destructive force of a shotgun is devastating. The bulk of the pellets penetrate the skin and underlying tissues as a relatively compact mass. As the discharge distance increases, so does the dispersal of the individual pellets. DiMaio[4] states that birdshot with a discharge distance of 2 ft causes a single entrance hole ¾ to 1 inch in diameter, and that at 3 ft this could be ⅞ to 1¼ inch with scalloped edges. By 4 ft the hole ranges from 1 to 1¾ inches with scattered pellets around the main hole (Fig. 8.10). A definite cuff of satellite holes forms with discharge distances of 6–7 ft and the central hole has an irregular outline. As the distance increases further, the central hole diminishes and the number of holes created by individual pellets increases.

It can be readily appreciated that considering the body size of the victim (e.g. goshawk) many of the diverging pellets will pass above, below, in front of, behind or to the sides of the target. In these circumstances it is generally impossible to give an accurate estimate of the discharge distance (the distance between the end of the barrel and the victim). Nevertheless, radiographs are helpful in providing guidance on whether the shot was 'distant' or 'close'. A wide distribution of pellets involving the body and legs of, say, a bird of prey (Fig. 8.11) indicates that the gun was discharged yards (metres) from the target. In contrast, a mass of pellets in relatively close contact with one another would suggest that the gun had been discharged no more than a few feet (1–2 metres) from the target (Fig. 8.12).

At distances of less than 1 ft (30 cm) soot deposits may be found on the hair or skin. Tattooing of the skin by powder is partially dependent on the type of powder but is

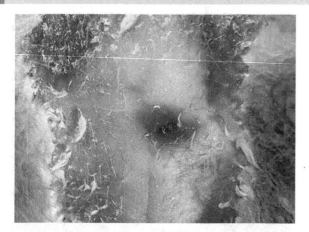

Fig. 8.13 – Entrance hole of a single shotgun pellet in the breast of a buzzard. Note surrounding bruising. This injury was not immediately fatal. The bird died from peritonitis later.

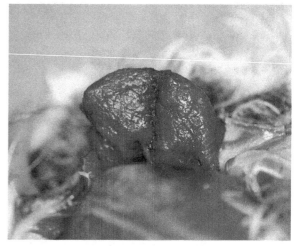

Fig. 8.15 – Shotgun pellet track through the pectoral muscle of a buzzard.

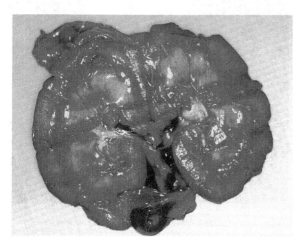

Fig. 8.14 – Tracks through dog kidney caused by shotgun pellets.

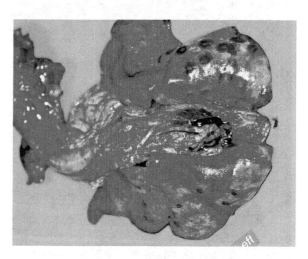

Fig. 8.16 – Non-fatal shotgun pellet injuries to the lungs of a male dog. Numerous pellets penetrated the right side of the dog, with many entering the right lung and mediastinum and a smaller number tracking into the left lung.

also influenced by the density of hair and feathers. Close-range shot may result in the wadding from the shotgun cartridge being embedded in the wound.

Entry holes of individual pellets are small, depending on the size of the pellets, and are frequently surrounded by a halo of bruising (Fig. 8.13). Pellet tracks are sometimes difficult to follow throughout their entire length but are often highlighted by ecchymotic haemorrhages and short haemorrhagic lines as they traverse vascular organs such as the lungs or kidneys (Fig. 8.14). In large muscles, clear pellet tracks can often be recognised (Fig. 8.15). Fatal injury depends on severe haemorrhage or major damage to vital organs. The results of distant shotgun wounding are unpredictable with, on occasion, rapidly fatal injury being caused by a single pellet whilst, in other circumstances, numerous shotgun pellets can penetrate the body cavities, striking organs such as the liver, kidneys, lungs and heart, and yet fail to kill (Fig. 8.16). This latter type of injury is a major

welfare issue with the animal suffering considerable pain and distress.

Subtle, non-fatal injuries caused by single shotgun pellets are readily overlooked but may provide vital evidence regarding the persecution of birds of prey (Fig. 8.17).

Exit holes caused by shotgun pellets are relatively uncommon in the thorax or abdomen of large mammals unless heavy ('buckshot') pellets were used. In small mammals and birds, exit holes do occur and tend to be of a similar size to, but less numerous than, the entry holes. Again, bruising may surround the exit wounds.

Perforating wounds of the avian skull may provide clear evidence of the direction of travel of the pellets (Fig. 8.18).

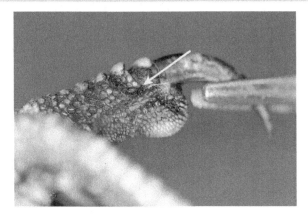

Fig. 8.17 – Single shotgun pellet injury to the toe of a buzzard. The pellet is embedded proximal to the talon (arrow). Bleeding is limited but the medial aspect of the toe is bruised.

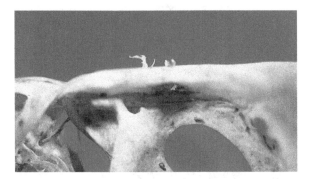

Fig. 8.18 – Exit hole of shotgun pellet through the skull above the eye of a hen harrier. The pellet entered from below and exited through the top of the head causing spicules of bone to be elevated.

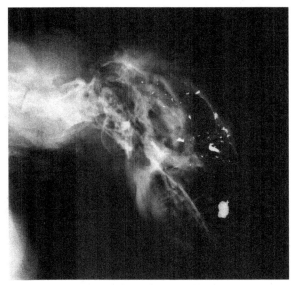

Fig. 8.19 – Adult badger shot in the head by a solid-nosed .22 bullet. A large fragment of bullet has lodged in the nasal cavity.

Rifle bullet wounds

Most, if not all, rifle bullet wounds likely to be encountered by veterinarians will be the result of 'intermediate' or 'distant' shots.[5] Even those shots used, for example, to kill snared or trapped animals are unlikely to be 'contact' wounds.

Rimfire

Entry holes of low-velocity .22 calibre bullets are small (3–5 mm in diameter). The shape of the entry hole is partially dependent on the angle at which the bullet strikes the skin. If the angle is perpendicular to the skin surface then the hole will be circular, whereas a tangential shot will cause an elliptical hole. Without clipping the hair, these wounds are difficult to find. The margin of the hole may show an abrasion ring caused as the bullet forced itself through the epidermis. Again, this abrasion ring may be circular or elliptical. Solid-nosed or hollow-nosed bullets that do not strike bone show limited deformity and may come to rest in soft tissues. (These bullets offer excellent opportunities for ballistics experts to match with suspect rifles.)

When the bullet strikes bone, the bullet is usually damaged, shedding fragments of metal, and the bone is fractured or splintered. Head shots cause multiple cranial fractures and fragmentation of the bullet and these fragments can be widely distributed in the brain, which is usually extensively damaged. Portions of bullet may exit the cranial cavity to become lodged in the nasal cavities, nasal sinuses and oral cavity, or embedded in the facial or neck muscles (Fig. 8.19).

Radiographs can provide the clue to the initially perplexing necropsy picture where no bullet is found at the end of the haemorrhagic suspect bullet track. Low-velocity .22 bullets may, as they lose energy, slip between and along the fascial planes in skeletal muscle. Thus, the final part of the bullet's path is obscure, and location of the bullet without the assistance of radiographs can be problematic. Similarly, .22 bullets may track subcutaneously in large birds (e.g. swan) to lodge under the skin on the opposite side of the body to the entry hole, leaving little or no trace of their passage (Fig. 8.20).

Rimfire bullets may cause perforating wounds to the abdomen leaving no radiographic evidence of passage of the bullet through the animal. If the bullet does not mushroom, the exit hole may be of a similar size to the entry wound. However, a greater degree of bruising surrounds the exit hole and the wound margins may be somewhat everted and lack an abrasion ring. Bleeding from the exit wound may be greater than from the entry wound.

Centrefire

Centrefire ammunition causes substantially different injuries compared with low-velocity rimfire bullets. The damage caused by a high-velocity bullet (defined as a bullet with a

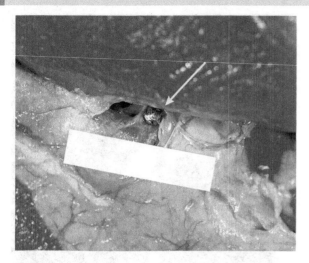

Fig. 8.20 – A .22 bullet lodged subcutaneously (arrow) on the right side of an adult swan. This bullet penetrated the skin on the left side of the body and travelled subcutaneously around the body and came to rest on the right side.

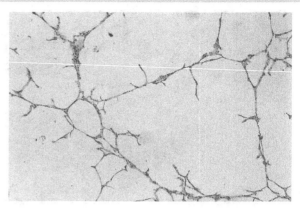

Fig. 8.22 – Red deer lung. Microscopic appearance of alveolar over-distension and alveolar septal rupture caused by the passage of a .270 bullet through the lung.

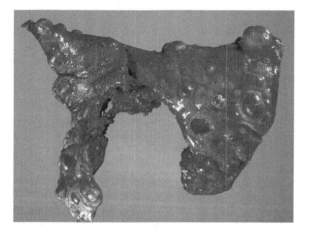

Fig. 8.21 – Roe deer lung (left side) showing destruction of the central area and extensive emphysematous bullae elsewhere, caused by a .243 bullet.

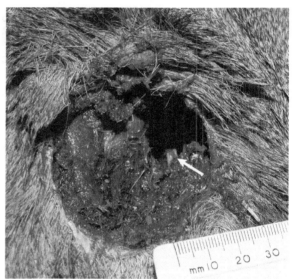

Fig. 8.23 – Roe deer chest. Exit hole of .243 bullet. Note fractured end of rib (arrow) and contamination of the wound by rumen contents.

muzzle velocity greater than 2000 fps) is not confined to the tissues penetrated by the bullet but extends to involve surrounding structures. This pattern of wounding is a consequence of the rapid transfer of kinetic energy from the bullet into the tissues causing the formation of a 'temporary cavity' within the tissues. The cavity created by centrefire hunting ammunition may extend to 30 times the diameter of the bullet before collapsing to form the permanent wound track. The temporary cavity results in stretching and devitalisation of the tissues, and affected organs may be partially or completely disintegrated. Hunting bullets are designed specifically to deform and to fragment, thereby ensuring rapid transfer of energy to the body and massive damage. Examples of gross and microscopic injuries caused by these bullets are shown in Figures 8.21 and 8.22.

The entry wound of centrefire ammunition may approximate to the diameter of the bullet, but care should be taken not to base any decisions on bullet calibre on the size of the entry hole. There are many variables such as the angle of strike, movement of the animal and the elasticity of the skin that can affect the shape and size of the entry hole.

Exit wounds reflect the extent of the deformation and fragmentation of the bullet together with additional injury caused by fragments of bone propelled out of the body by the force of the impact. These wounds are larger than the entry wounds. The wound margins are irregular and portions of internal organs, stomach contents, fragments of ribs or spine, and blood may contaminate the surrounding hair (Fig. 8.23).

Birds are, from time to time, shot with high-velocity bullets. Avian bones are generally of light structure and

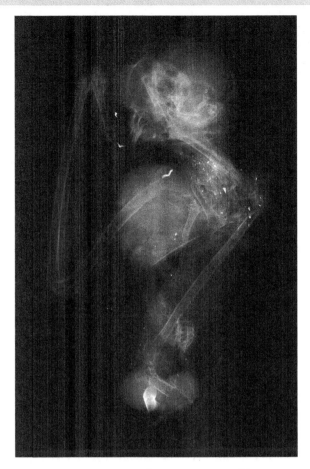

Fig. 8.24 – Radiograph of an owl (with perforating wound) showing fragments of radio-opaque material. The 'flying seagull' shaped fragments are portions of the disrupted copper jacket of a high-velocity rifle bullet.

offer limited resistance to the passage of such bullets. Perforating wounds are, therefore, common and the entry and exit wounds may be of similar size. Nevertheless, study of radiographs of such cases may show fragments of metal in the wound track (Fig. 8.24).

Multiple gunshot wounds and post-mortem injuries

Animals may be non-fatally wounded by high-velocity bullets and one or more subsequent shots are required to administer the *coup de grace*. The fatal shot is usually the final one, but care needs to be taken to separate ante-mortem from post-mortem gunshot injuries. The lack of significant bleeding along a permanent wound track is often the main feature that indicates that a shot was administered after death (Case study 8.1, Figs 8.25 & 8.26).

A combination of radiography and careful post-mortem examination will assist in the detection of fraudulent insurance claims such as the horse that is euthanased following fracture of the leg and is subsequently shot in the leg, after death, in an attempt to falsify the evidence related to the initial accident.

Care of pellets and bullets found at post-mortem examination

Matching of rifling marks on bullets and air-rifle pellets, or determination of the composition of shotgun pellets, falls within the remit of the ballistics experts. However, careless handling of bullets and pellets by the pathologist, at the time they are removed from the body, can obscure vital marks. It is important to adopt a standard procedure that will ensure that no damage to the bullets or pellets occurs during the retrieval process or during transport of the specimens to the ballistics laboratory:

Case study 8.1

A pine marten recovered from a domestic freezer showed two major areas of injury. The first involved extensive blood staining over both sides of the chest. An 8-mm hole was present low on the right side of the chest close to the breast bone. In the left chest wall, between ribs 4 and 5, was a 12 × 5-mm irregular hole. Massive haemorrhage had occurred into both sides of the chest cavity. The lower parts of the middle areas of both left and right lungs showed extensive destruction.

The second was an elliptical hole (6 × 4 mm) on the top of the head, into which hair had been pulled. The skin surrounding this hole was haemorrhagic over a poorly defined area measuring 40 × 35 mm. A 6-mm diameter hole was present in the skull. Alongside this hole was an irregular opening in the skull caused

by separation of fractures of the cranium. The floor and wall of the left side of the skull was fractured in numerous places and a large irregular hole (17 × 14 mm) was present in the left side of the face at the angle of the jaw. The majority of the brain was destroyed. Fragments of bullet were present in the head, jaw, and in the skin at the angle of the jaw. There was no evidence of significant haemorrhage along the track of this bullet wound from the top of the head to the left side of the face.

It was concluded that the pine marten was killed by a perforating rifle bullet injury to the chest (Fig. 8.25) and that a second shot was administered to the head shortly after death (Fig. 8.26).

Case study 8.1 (continued)

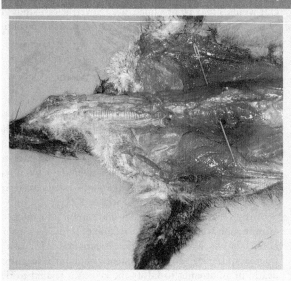

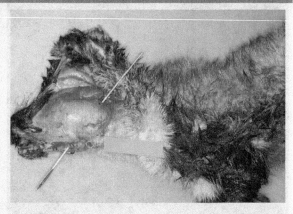

Fig. 8.26 – Pine marten shown in Figure 8.25. A second bullet passed through the head from top to left side of the face shortly after death. Note lack of haemorrhage.

Fig. 8.25 – Pine marten fatally wounded in the chest by a bullet that entered the right side and exited close to the left shoulder. The metal probe indicates the track of the bullet.

- Pellets or bullets should be located accurately by reference to radiographs taken in two planes.
- Careful dissection in the vicinity of the object should allow the pathologist to feel the metal fragments. All contact between the scalpel blade and the metal object should be avoided.
- Gently separate and remove the soft tissues surrounding the pellet or bullet.
- Using fingers or gauze-covered forceps, place the pellet or bullet in a small plastic bowl.
- Wash gently in water to remove blood and any strands of tissue that are adhering to the irregular surface of the object.
- Remove the bullet from the water and dip in 70% alcohol to help dispel any remaining water droplets.
- Air-dry and wrap in 'bubble-wrap' or similar material that is transparent and soft. Avoid cotton wool and other such materials that become snagged on the surface of the specimen.

- Place the wrapped specimen in a clear plastic specimen bottle with sufficient wrapping material to prevent the specimen rattling about in the container.
- Seal, identify, sign and date the container.

References

1. Thomas G. Modern guns. In: Brown N, ed. Shotguns and cartridges for game and clays, 5th edn. London: A & C Black; 1987:17–35.
2. Marshall–Ball R. The sporting rifle: a user's handbook. Shrewsbury: Swan Hill Press; 1995.
3. Smith WD. Air rifle ammunition and its influence on wounding potential. Arch Emerg Med 1985; 2:25–29.
4. DiMaio VJM. Wounds from shotguns. In: Gunshot wounds, 2nd edn. Boca Raton: CRC Press; 1999:203–252.
5. DiMaio VJM. An introduction to the classification of gunshot wounds. In: Gunshot wounds, 2nd edn. Boca Raton: CRC Press; 1999:65–122.

9 | Asphyxia and Drowning

Introduction

The term asphyxia covers a number of conditions that result in interference with uptake and utilisation of oxygen and elimination of carbon dioxide.

Asphyxia can be caused by:

- Lack of oxygen in the inspired air
- Obstruction of the air passages
- Restriction of chest movements
- Histotoxic anoxia.

Words that are commonly used in asphyxia cases include suffocation, smothering, strangulation, choking, throttling, hanging and crush asphyxia.

General features

Asphyxiation may occur under a variety of circumstances ranging from non-accidental injury in the form of hanging or smothering, through poisoning with cyanide, to death during unsuitable transportation. Additionally, accidental asphyxiation arises in house fires and in farmyard incidents such as postural asphyxiation where a bull, for example, falls in a handling crush and the trachea is occluded as the neck is twisted to the side or under the body. The final cause of death in all of these incidents is considered to be cerebral hypoxia followed by cardiac arrest.

The time taken for unconsciousness to supervene and for death to occur is frequently difficult to assess. Sudden, complete and simultaneous occlusion of both carotids will lead to unconsciousness in a number of seconds. However, this is an unusual event and in most cases of asphyxiation unconsciousness is preceded by a period of intense distress as the animal fights for its life. Struggling during asphyxiation of a conscious animal may lead to bruising on face, legs, hips and spine that should not be confused with other causes of trauma.

Strangulation

Strangulation may be deliberate or accidental. Canine victims of deliberate strangulation may be hanged from a tree branch (Fig. 9.1), a loft hatch or other convenient high point. The dog's lead, rope, dressing-gown cord, electric flex or wire may be used. Accidental strangulation can occur when a tethered dog jumps over, or on to, a kennel roof or platform and becomes trapped with the tether tight around the neck. In horses and ponies, accidental strangu-

lation by a neck rope or head collar can result from poor animal husbandry practices. Similarly, non-elasticated collars can contribute to strangulation of domestic cats.

Externally there may be limited evidence of ligature marks in fatal strangulation. The hair and looseness of the skin around the neck can protect against skin abrasion (Case study 9.1). However, careful examination may reveal areas where there is indentation of hair (Fig. 9.2) or patchy loss of hair or reddening or mild bruising of the skin (Fig. 9.3). Cyanosis may affect the teats, perineum and vulva. Focal intradermal haemorrhages can develop in the skin of the posterior abdomen and immediately cranial to the ventral vulva in dogs that have been hanged. There may be more generalised congestion of the skin of the ventral neck, thorax or abdomen.

Subcutaneous bruising may be present over the larynx, at the angle of the jaw (Fig. 9.4) or where the knot in the ligature has tightened against the neck in animals that have been hanged by being dropped from a height. These animals may also show epiglottic congestion, fresh ecchymotic haemorrhages over the laryngeal cartilages or in the glosso-epiglottic fold and congestion of the sclera of one or both eyes. Fracture of the hyoid apparatus may occur in mature animals with mineralised hyoid bones (Fig. 9.5). There appears to be limited published information on the age of mineralisation of the hyoid bones[1] in the various species and breeds, and radiographic examination of the neck in alleged strangulation cases is recommended before the commencement of the necropsy.

Froth, usually pink in colour, is commonly found in the lower trachea. This froth may extend into the larynx, although in most cases it collects in the lower to mid trachea.

Careful examination of the lungs is essential. Grossly, they are congested, sometimes severely, and show irregular areas of collapse, giving the surface an uneven appearance. As might be expected, the diaphragmatic lobes, which are the most dependent lobes when the animal is hanging, show the greatest congestion. In some cases the lungs are over-inflated and rib markings are clearly defined. Histologically, a combination of areas of alveolar over-distension, recent intra-alveolar haemorrhage and alveolar flooding with pink-staining fluid is the characteristic picture. Free blood within bronchi and bronchioles may also be a feature. Absence of a significant inflammatory cell response in the interstitium or alveolar lumina is an important differential observation.

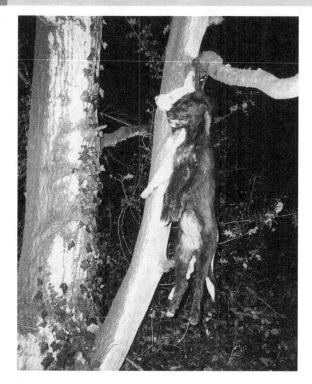

Fig. 9.1 – Two puppies hanged from a tree by their leads. (By kind permission of the Royal Society for the Prevention of Cruelty to Animals.)

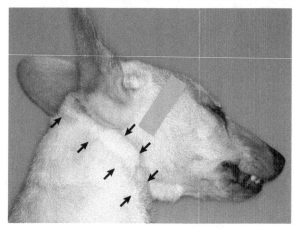

Fig. 9.2 – The lighter coloured puppy shown in Figure 9.1 has indentation of the hair around the neck (arrows) but no abrasions of skin or neck bruising.

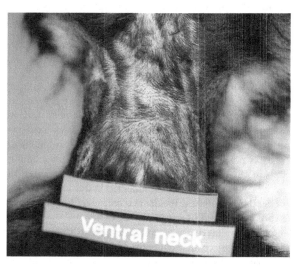

Fig. 9.3 – The darker puppy shown in Figure 9.1 had mild bruising and reddening of the skin on the ventral surface and both sides of the neck. It was necessary to clip the hair to appreciate this change.

Case study 9.1

Fire fighters attended a fire in an apartment. The blaze, which was centred on the bedroom, was extinguished and the remainder of the apartment was searched for victims or other signs of fire. In the kitchen, a middle-aged female dog, 'Taffy', was found lying in her bed. She was dead.

The circumstances of the fire raised suspicions of arson and the police requested that the body of the dog be subjected to post-mortem examination to confirm the cause of death, suspected to be smoke inhalation.

The dog was in excellent bodily condition, was clearly well looked after and showed no signs of natural disease. A single subcutaneous bruise, measuring 45 × 30 mm was present on the back of the neck. The lungs, windpipe, larynx, eyes and subcutaneous tissues were extensively congested and evidence of smoke inhalation was absent. This combination of findings suggested that Taffy had died as a result of asphyxiation by ligature rather than smoke inhalation.

During interview by the police, the boyfriend of the dog's owner admitted hanging Taffy by the cord of a dressing gown from the loft hatch before setting the apartment alight.

The pathophysiology of the pulmonary congestion and oedema is not entirely clear,[2,3] but is believed to involve a combination of changes including:

- alterations in hydrostatic pressures related to negative intrathoracic pressure caused by inspiration against an obstruction in the upper respiratory tract
- increased left ventricular afterload
- pooling of blood in the pulmonary capillaries following massive sympathetic outflow.

Neurogenic factors, possibly associated with hypoxia, may also have a role. It is important that a thorough check for

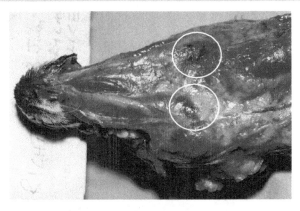

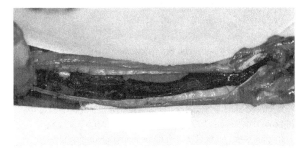

Fig. 9.6 – An adult female dog buried alive showed extensive inhalation of mud into the windpipe and main bronchi.

Fig. 9.4 – A middle-aged female dog was hanged by her lead in the stairwell of a block of apartments. She was rescued quickly but was dead when released. Note bruising caused by the tightened collar at angles of jaw (circles). Haemorrhage was also present on the left side of the larynx and in the glosso-epiglottic fold.

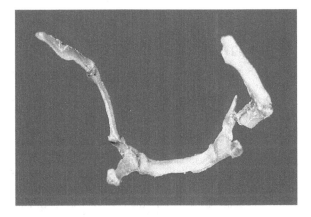

Fig. 9.5 – Fractured hyoid bone from an adult badger who died from strangulation in a wire snare.

natural disease of the upper respiratory tract is undertaken, as there is evidence that pulmonary oedema can be secondary to laryngeal pathology.[4]

Choking and smothering

Choking refers to blockage of the upper airways by a foreign body. This could have an accidental cause such as inhalation of a small ball or other object during play. It also occurs following non-accidental live burial that results in inhalation of ground, mud, sand or other material in which the animal was buried (Fig. 9.6). Such materials can enter the mouth after death, but penetration of the nasal cavities or the trachea indicates a distinct respiratory effort by a live animal rather than passive seepage in a cadaver. Exceptions to this general rule may occur when dead animals are buried in catastrophic events such as landslides or earthquakes where great forces are in play and mud may

be forced into the air passages of animals that died from other causes.

Severe injury to the head and face may result in fatal obstruction of the air passages (see Chapter 6: Wounds and injuries, Case 6.5, Fig. 6.16). Additionally, inhalation of blood from damaged turbinates, hard palate, nasal bones or base of skull fractures can obstruct the trachea and lower airways, leading to fatal choking. Similarly, throat cuts that enter the trachea can lead to choking on inhaled blood.

The pulmonary pathology of choking is characterised by congestion, intra-alveolar flooding and haemorrhage, and alveolar over-distension. Portions of the material that caused the choking may be found in the bronchi and, if the particles are sufficiently small and the respiratory efforts sufficient, in the alveolar lumina.

Smothering of domestic animals by closure of the mouth and nostrils may be accompanied by a variable distribution of tell-tale bruising under the chin, over the premaxilla, maxillary and frontal bones, and on the inner aspects of the lips where they are in contact with the teeth (or dental pad in ruminants). The pulmonary changes are similar to those in fatal strangulations.

Obstruction of airflow may also result from blunt trauma to the neck/thorax which results in hyperextension of the neck, stretching of the trachea and avulsion of the trachea within the anterior thorax, cranial to the bifurcation. Dyspnoea following tracheal avulsion may have a rapid onset or develop days or weeks after the traumatic incident.[5] Such injuries can occur in, for example, road traffic accidents or from non-accidental injury (Case study 9.2).

Suffocation and crush asphyxia

Transportation of wildlife in unsuitable containers can lead to suffocation of some, or all, of the consignment. Pulmonary congestion and oedema in the absence of natural disease provides useful corroborating evidence when wildlife law enforcement agencies are investigating illegal or substandard transportation.

Deaths of livestock during transportation in hot weather result from a variable combination of hyperthermia, smothering and crush asphyxia. Crush asphyxia refers to death

> **Case study 9.2**
>
> The owner of three small kittens claimed to the police that her ex-partner had assaulted her and 'broke the necks' of two of the kittens.
>
> Post-mortem examination showed one kitten to have a fractured skull and haemorrhage over the posterior part of the brain. The second kitten showed avulsion of the trachea (i.e. forcible separation of the windpipe from the lungs a short distance in front of the lungs) and haemorrhage into the chest cavity. Bruises over the side of the head and in the upper part of the neck suggested that the kitten may have been gripped around the head whilst the neck was over-extended.

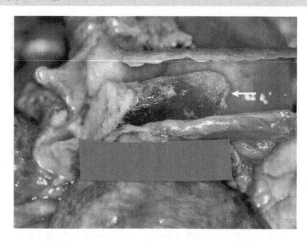

Fig. 9.7 – This elderly male dog was found dead, partially submerged in a stream and, after an incomplete initial post-mortem examination, his body was frozen. A second post-mortem examination revealed frozen stable foam (arrow) in the windpipe and bronchi.

caused by restriction of the chest movements by the weight of bodies or other heavy objects pressed against the victim.

Poisonous gases

Carbon monoxide produced by faulty domestic heaters or from car exhaust fumes is rapidly absorbed through the lungs and leads to the formation of carboxyhaemoglobin. In fatal cases the oxygen-carrying capacity of the blood is reduced to the point where death occurs from anoxia.

Carboxyhaemoglobin is relatively stable and, at necropsy, the mucous membranes and internal organs may appear unusually pink in colour. Where the cadaver has been frozen and then thawed before necropsy, care needs to be taken not to confuse the diffuse pinkness commonly found in such bodies with the changes induced by carbon monoxide poisoning. In some dogs poisoned by car exhaust fumes there is generalised dark congestion of the mucous membranes including unusual injection of the uterine cervix.

Cyanide poisoning of badgers and other wildlife can be difficult to prove. There may be circumstantial evidence of use of cyanide-containing poisons in the vicinity of the animals, but detection of cyanide in cadavers that have been dead for some time before discovery may be unsuccessful. In theory, cyanide poisoning results in bright red coloration of the organs. However, as post-mortem changes develop, the abnormal colour fades and the absence of the characteristic colour change should not automatically discount the possibility of fatal cyanide intoxication. In fresher cadavers, the smell of bitter almond may be a useful indicator of cyanide. In any suspect case, the pathologist should exercise care during the necropsy to avoid inhaling released gases, which may contain toxic quantities of cyanide.

Smoke inhalation

Examination of cases where smoke inhalation is a possibility requires slight changes to normal necropsy protocols (see Protocol A in Chapter 7: Thermal injuries, p 51).

Drowning

Although it seems obvious, it is worth noting that the coat of most drowned animals is wet when they are first presented for examination. In non-accidental drowning of companion animals, the perpetrator may attempt to dry the coat with a towel before taking the animal to the veterinary surgery. However, the deeper parts of the coat, particularly in thick-coated dogs, remain damp.

In what appears, at first sight, to be a clear case of drowning (e.g. a dog is recovered from a river with a heavy weight attached by a rope to the neck or with both hind and forelimbs firmly tied together) it is important that other causes of death are eliminated.

Congestion of the lungs and variable quantities of pink frothy fluid in the bronchi and the trachea are consistent features (Fig. 9.7). Froth is thought to arise as a result of rapid respiratory movements agitating inhaled water in the airways and mixing the water with respiratory tract mucus and surfactant. The longer the duration of the respiratory efforts, the greater is the potential for the formation of stable froth. An animal that is immersed and allowed to surface several times before finally dying may have more airway froth than one that dies rapidly following initial inhalation of water.

Drowning may result in non-specific histopathological changes. However, the presence of plant material, mud or sand in the distal airways is highly significant. Although such matter may enter the upper respiratory tract after death, the length of the windpipe (in most animals) makes it unlikely that it will migrate passively to the level of the smaller airways in reasonably fresh cadavers. Drowned animals may show alveolar over-distension, attenuation of alveolar septa, narrowing of alveolar capillaries, alveolar rupture, intra-alveolar haemorrhage and flooding by pale fluid. Nevertheless, no single histopathological change is diagnostic of drowning and it is the combination of the history, gross appearance and histopathological changes that may assist in the differentiation of drowning from immersion shortly after death.[6] If the water in which the animal was immersed was heavily contaminated with bacteria, histopathological examination will show widespread bacterial colonisation of the lungs in the absence of an inflammatory response. It needs to be accepted that, in most cases, a diagnosis of drowning will depend on the exclusion of other causes of death.

Newborn kittens or puppies have limited ability to struggle, but bigger or stronger animals make determined efforts to survive. Forcible drowning can occur in two ways: by pressing and holding the head or whole animal under the water, or by holding the animal upside down by the legs before lowering the creature into the water to submerge the head. Bruising is a common feature in animals forcibly immersed in baths, basins or other suitable receptacles. In the first method of drowning, bruising develops over the side of the neck and the back where the animal was gripped, or occurs over bony prominences, such as the spine of the scapula or the facial crest where the animal was pressed against the bottom of the vessel. When held by the legs and inverted, bruising may be found on the distal limbs where the legs were gripped or tied together (Fig. 9.8).

Sea mammals trapped in nets die from asphyxia related to the closure of the glottis. Usually, water is not inhaled, as in terrestrial mammals, and the formation of froth by rapid respiratory movements agitating inhaled water in the trachea is not a feature of 'dry drowning' of sea mammals. Many seals and porpoises drowned in fishing nets show skin wounds caused during the struggle to escape.

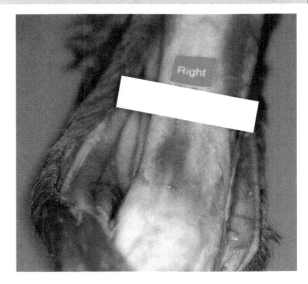

Fig. 9.8 – Dog (as in Fig. 9.7). Bruising of the lower forelimbs suggests that this dog may have been restrained just above the wrists (carpi).

References

1. Fox MW. Developmental physiology and behaviour. In: Canine pediatrics. Springfield: Charles C Thomas; 1966:25–29.

2. Myers NC, Walls RE. Pathophysiologic mechanisms of non-cardiogenic pulmonary edema. *J* Am Vet Med Assoc 1995; 207:1018–1019.

3. Drobatz KJ, Saunders HM. Noncardiogenic pulmonary edema. In: Current veterinary therapy. XIII: Small animal practice. Philadelphia: W B Saunders; 2000:810–812.

4. Kelly LY. Pulmonary edema secondary to upper airway obstruction in the dog. J Am Anim Hosp Assoc 1989; 25:207–212.

5. White RN, Burton CA. Surgical management of intrathoracic tracheal avulsion in cats: long-term results in 9 consecutive cases. Vet Surg 2000; 29:430–435.

6. Reidbord HE. Drowning. In: Perper JA, Wecht CH, eds. Microscopic diagnosis in forensic pathology. Springfield: Charles C Thomas; 1980:206–210.

10 | Injuries Associated with Physical Agents

Hyperthermia/heat stroke

Heat stroke is a result of exposure to a hot environment where the normal physiological mechanisms, used to maintain the core body temperature within defined limits, are overwhelmed and the animal is unable to prevent its body heat rising to harmful and frequently fatal levels. Considerable investigation of the pathophysiology and circumstances predisposing to heat stroke has been undertaken.[1-8] The typical heatstroke patient is usually collapsed, has a very high body temperature, and shows serious complications in the brain, kidney, liver and circulation. Veterinarians may be asked to examine a variety of animals affected by heat stroke, including horses, cattle and pigs, but dogs appear to be the subject of forensic investigations more commonly than other species.

The average normal rectal temperature of a dog is 102°F (38.9°C). During hyperthermia the core body temperature rises, and when it exceeds 106°F (41°C) death may supervene. The upper fatal body temperature in dogs is considered to be 107.6°F (42°C).

Some 73% of heat from dogs is lost through radiation and conduction from the body surface to the surrounding air. The bulk of the remaining heat is lost by evaporation from the tongue and upper respiratory tract during panting. Loss of heat by evaporation is greatly affected by the relative humidity. Consequently, in environments where high ambient temperature is combined with high relative humidity, dogs are in constant danger of being unable to keep their body temperature within the normal physiological range.

This type of scenario can readily occur inside a vehicle in summer. As the temperature rises in the vehicle, the dog pants to cool down but the fluid lost via evaporation from the mouth causes the relative humidity to rise inside the vehicle. The dog's body temperature rises and the dog becomes restless, thereby increasing heat generation in the muscles and putting further strain on the already overburdened heat regulatory mechanisms. If ventilation in the vehicle is insufficient to remove the water-laden air from around the dog in the vehicle, the situation deteriorates progressively. The time taken to develop clinical and pathological features of heat stroke/hyperthermia is variable depending on the environmental conditions (ambient temperature, humidity, ventilation) and to some extent on the coping mechanisms of the individual dog. It may range from less than an hour in extreme cases to several hours in less severe circumstances (Case study 10.1, Fig. 10.1).

All organs (including the mucous membranes, which may be discoloured deeply red or dirty brown) are affected by vascular congestion. This change is most pronounced in the trachea (Fig. 10.2), lungs and bronchi. The heart, kidneys, meninges, lymph nodes and muscles may also show severe congestion.[9]

The speed of onset of rigor mortis is increased by high environmental and body temperatures and muscular effort.[10] For all of these reasons, the onset of rigor mortis in dogs that die from heat stroke can be extremely rapid. The rate of post-mortem changes is also accelerated in hyperthermic animals.

Frostbite

In small animals, the ears, digits, scrotum and tip of tail are the areas most commonly affected because of their peripheral position, lack of hair or limited blood supply.[11] The hind feet of calves are vulnerable, together with the tips of the ears and the distal 5–10 cm of the tail. Calves that are unwell as a consequence of pneumonia, diarrhoea or other systemic infections are at greater risk than healthy calves.[12,13] Adult cattle may develop frostbite of the teats, base of udder and scrotum.

Frozen areas may develop a dark or bluish appearance with diffuse subcutaneous oedema and haemorrhage. Ischaemic necrosis may lead to sloughing, but the extent of the damage may not be fully demarcated until 4–15 days after the incident.[14,15]

Frostbite in birds is not uncommon[16] and usually affects the feet, although distal wing necrosis of falcons may also be a cold-related injury.[17] In addition to lack of acclimatisation of non-native birds, various risk factors include unseasonable weather, anaesthesia, wire cages, metal leg bands and any constrictions to blood supply, such as over-tight bandaging or previous injury. The scaly legs of birds do not blister, as might be seen in mammals, but oedema of the foot or lower limb may be noted after 24 hours. It may take 3–6 weeks before demarcation of viable and dead tissue can be appreciated visually.

Electrocution

Injuries caused by electricity range from electrothermal burns through fractures, cardiac and neurological damage,

Case study 10.1

Two adult black Labrador dogs were confined in a vehicle in full sun on a hot summer's afternoon. The windows were left open approximately 2–3 inches (5–7 cm). About 2.5 hours later, one dog was found dead (Fig. 10.1) and the other in deep distress. Fully developed rigor mortis was demonstrated by the attending veterinarian 50 minutes after the vehicle was opened, but may have been present earlier.

Post-mortem examination showed the characteristic features of heatstroke, including brown–red discoloration of the lining of the mouth and extreme congestion of the conjunctivae, subcutaneous tissues, lining of the windpipe and all internal organs. Post-mortem change was advanced.

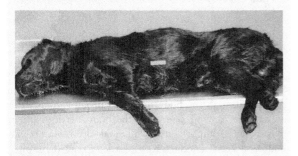

Fig. 10.1 – This Labrador dog died from hyperthermia after being left in a motor vehicle (see Case study 10.1). Note blood-stained fluid on the table under the chin. This has leaked from the mouth and nose.

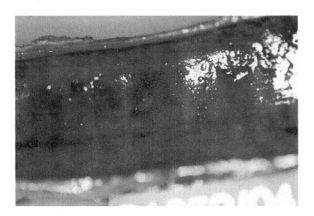

Fig. 10.2 – Labrador (see Case study 10.1). The lining of the windpipe shows marked congestion.

vascular and other tissue damage to death. Considerable information is available on the mechanisms, immediate effects, long-term deficits and causes of death in humans.[18] The nature of the injuries caused by the passage of the current is governed by the physics related to the flow of the electrical charge. Therefore, many of the observations made on people may be directly applicable to domestic

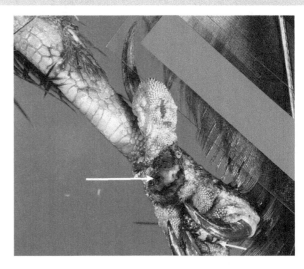

Fig. 10.3 – Buzzard. This deep burn on the foot was caused by contact with a high-voltage electricity cable. Note exposed bone (white arrow) and scavenging beetle (yellow arrow).

animals. However, some differences related to posture and gait are clearly present.

Electrothermal burns

Electrical current, measured in amperes, is the 'energy' that flows through a conductor and is responsible for the generation of heat (heat generated is proportional to the amperage squared). The current flows from one contact point to another and it is at these points of contact that the greatest tissue damage often occurs. Injury to deeper organs can be patchy and unpredictable, with burned tissue lying adjacent to unharmed tissues. As a general principle, the longer the contact with a high-voltage current, the greater will be the generation of heat and destruction of tissue.

Burns to the lips and mouth of domestic animals (e.g. puppies and hamsters) may be caused by chewing through the insulation of live electricity cables in the home. Such burns are usually less severe than the injuries associated with high-voltage cables.

When skin and hair are dry and electrical resistance is high, more heat is generated and the likelihood of burns and hair singeing is increased.

Wildlife can suffer very severe burns when they contact high-voltage electricity cables. Prolonged (seconds) contact causes full-thickness skin burns and destruction of underlying tissues including muscle, tendons and bone (Fig. 10.3). The skin at the margins of the burns may be carbonised and the surrounding skin or feathers may be coated with soft, brown crumbly material, which is the remnant of heated blood/tissue (Fig. 10.4). Severe burning may also happen when indirect contact is established in the form of an electrical arc between two objects of differing potential.

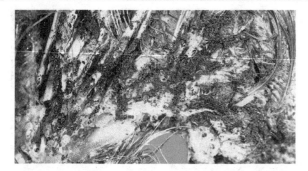

Fig. 10.4 – Buzzard (same bird as in Fig. 10.3). A severe burn was present on the leading edge of the left wing. Note the coating of brown material on the skin and feathers. This is the remnant of heated blood/tissue.

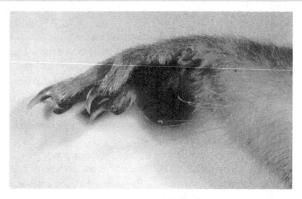

Fig. 10.6 – Squirrel (same animal as in Fig. 10.5). Hair was also singed over the chest and along the forelegs. Note heat twisting of the longer hair close to the foot.

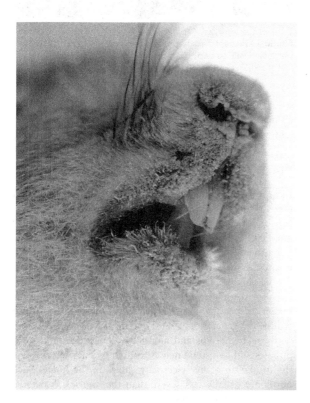

Fig. 10.5 – Squirrel. Singeing of hair around the mouth and nose was caused by an electrical flash that passed over the body and head.

Mechanism of death

Fatal electrocution is usually a result of the current passing through the body or head causing cardiac arrest or damage to vital centres in the brain. 'Stride voltage' may play an important role in fatal electrocution. The body is a better conductor of electricity than the ground. Consequently, when an electrical current is running through the ground, it will preferentially enter the body usually through one foot, exiting through another. The foot closer to the electrical source has a potential difference with the other feet, and the greater the potential difference the greater the risk to the animal. Large animals, such as cattle and horses, because of the distance between front and hind feet, are at particular risk from the effects of 'stride voltage'.[19]

Post-mortem findings

It is generally agreed that rigor mortis develops quickly and passes off early in electrocuted animals,[12,20] and is accompanied by accelerated post-mortem decomposition. Congestion and petechiae may occur throughout the body. This may be particularly noticeable in the upper respiratory tract, with linear tracheal haemorrhages being present. The blood may be dark and unclotted.

In pigs, muscular spasm following accidental electrocution may result in fractures of lumbosacral vertebrae, pelvis and femur.[21] Haemorrhage is associated with these injuries but careful post-mortem examination is required to reveal the extent of the pelvic injuries.

Some cadavers will have few indications of the cause of death and a diagnosis of electrocution will rely on exclusion of other causes, e.g. life-threatening acute infectious disease or chemical poisoning, and on other evidence such as clear indication of 'sudden' death (food in mouth) or confirmation of an electrical fault.

The temperature of an electrical arc is around 2500°C and causes deep burns at the point of contact.

Indirect contact can also be established as an electrical flash that splashes across the body rather than in the form of a defined arc. Electrical flashes may result in hair singeing and splash burns over a larger part of the body, but the burns are much less severe (Figs 10.5 & 10.6).

Lightning

Important differences exist between lightning strike and electrocution by artificial electricity. The duration of a lightning strike is extremely short and much of the strike washes over the outside of the body rather than passing through the internal organs. Deep burning is not a regular feature of lightning strike, although some singeing and superficial burns may be found. Linear burns on the medial aspects of the limbs are more commonly found than elsewhere on the body.[20] The 'arboreal' burn or 'feathering' marks on the skin are not true burns but rather a pattern of superficial injury caused by the electron shower induced by the lightning.[18] These marks are important findings and are most readily appreciated by reflection of the skin.

The effects of lightning strike vary and depend on whether the animal received a direct hit or suffered shock from spread through the ground or through direct or indirect contact with a conductor such as a fence.

Lightning strike close to the head may cause major damage as the electricity enters the body via the eyes, ears and mouth. More commonly, death is a consequence of cardiac arrest and neurological injury following spread of electricity through the earth or tree roots, entering the body via the feet. Animals resting against, or close to, a fence or pole may suffer flashover as the lightning jumps from the primary object on to the animal and then to the ground.

Many insurance claims for 'sudden death' in livestock are ascribed to lightning strike, but the veterinarian should investigate each of such claims thoroughly before reaching a conclusion. Various factors may need to be considered including:

- Were the animals moved after death but before the start of the veterinary investigation?
- Is it possible that they died at another locus and were relocated (e.g. next to a wire fence) in an attempt to give the impression that death was by lightning strike?
- Do local meteorology records provide information on lightning activity at the appropriate time?
- Is physical damage related to lightning strike (e.g. burnt or split trees or fences) present at the locus?
- Do the post-mortem signs support or undermine a diagnosis of lightning strike?
- Can an alternative cause of death be confirmed?

Chemical burns

Chemical burns are, in essence, severe manifestations of irritant contact dermatitis. In contrast to some other irritants (e.g. soaps, detergents and disinfectants), alkalis and acids may damage the skin immediately[11] but, like all irritant chemicals, the severity of the damage is influenced by the concentration of the substance and the duration of contact with the skin.

Distribution of lesions can be informative, with those on the feet, ventral abdomen and scrotum suggesting that the animal may have walked through, or been lying in, the irritant. Lesions on the back raise the possibility that the substance had been poured or splashed on to the animal. Chemical injury to the mouth may follow licking of material from elsewhere on the body.

Corneal damage may be caused by a variety of substances including *'bleaches, insecticides, shampoos and surgical skin preparations'*.[22] Alkalis are of particular concern, because they are able to penetrate all layers of the eye and may cause irreversible damage.

References

1. Drobatz KJ, Macintire DK. Heat induced illness in dogs: 42 cases (1976–1993). J Am Vet Med Assoc 1996; 209:1894–1899.
2. Gregory NG, Constantine E. Hyperthermia in dogs left in cars. Vet Rec 1996; 139:349–350.
3. Hanneman GD, Higgins EA, Price GT et al. Transient and permanent effects of hyperthermia in dogs: a study of a simulated air transport environmental stress. Am J Vet Res 1977; 38:955–958.
4. Holloway SA. Heatstroke in dogs. Compendium on Continuing Education for the Practicing Veterinarian 1992; 14:1598–1604.
5. Johnson K. Pathophysiology of heatstroke. Compendium on Continuing Education for the Practicing Veterinarian 1982; 4:141–144.
6. Krum SH, Osborne CA. Heatstroke in the dog: a polysystemic disorder. J Am Vet Med Assoc 1977; 170:531–535.
7. Larson RL, Carithers RW, Carithers BS. A review of heatstroke and its complications in the canine. N Z Vet J 1985; 33:202–206.
8. Ruslander D. Heatstroke. In: Kirk RW, Bonagura JD, eds. Kirk's current veterinary therapy, 11th edn. London: Saunders; 1992:143–146.
9. Ringler DJ. Inflammation and repair. In: Jones TC, Hunt RD, King NW, eds. Veterinary pathology, 6th edn. Baltimore: Williams & Wilkins; 1997:113–157.
10. Hulland TJ. Muscle and tendon. In: Jubb KVF, Kennedy PC, Palmer N, eds. Pathology of domestic animals, 4th edn, vol 1. San Diego: Academic Press; 1993:183–265.
11. Scott DW, Miller WH, Griffin CE. Environmental skin diseases. In: Muller and Kirk's small animal dermatology, 6th edn. Philadelphia: Saunders; 2001:1073–1111.
12. Radostits OM, Gay CC, Hinchcliff KW et al. Diseases associated with physical agents. In: Veterinary medicine, 10th edn. Edinburgh: Saunders Elsevier; 2007:1785–1795.
13. Cruz AM, Naylor JM. A retrospective study of frostbite injuries in calves (1982–1991). Can Vet J 1993; 34:306–308.
14. Yager JA, Scott DW. Skin and appendages. In: Jubb KVF, Kennedy PC, Palmer N, eds. Pathology of domestic animals, 4th edn, vol 1. San Diego: Academic Press; 1993:531–738.
15. Dhupa N. Hypothermia and frostbite. In: Morgan RV, Bright RM, Swartout MS, eds. Handbook of small animal practice, 4th edn. London: Saunders; 2003:1263–1265.
16. Wellehan JFX. Frostbite in birds: pathophysiology and treatment. Compendium on Continuing Education for the Practicing Veterinarian 2003; 25:776–781.
17. Forbes NA, Harcourt-Brown NH. Wing tip oedema and dry gangrene of raptors. Vet Rec 1991; 128:575–576.

18. Price T, Cooper MA. Electrical and lightning injuries. In: Rosen's emergency medicine: concepts and clinical practices, 5th edn, vol 3. St Louis: Mosby; 2002:2010–2020.

19. Novales M, Hermandez E, Lucena R. Electrocution in the horse. Vet Rec 1998; 142:68.

20. Anon. Lightning stroke and electrocution: introduction. In: Kahn CM, ed. The Merck veterinary manual. Whitehouse Stations, NJ: Merck; 2005:529–530.

21. Bildfell RJ, Camat BD, Lister DB. Posterior paralysis and electrocution of swine caused by accidental electric shock. J Vet Invest 1991; 3, 364–367.

22. Barnett KC, Crispin SA. Ocular emergencies and trauma. In: Feline ophthalmology: an atlas and text. Edinburgh: Elsevier Science; 2001:17–33.

11 | Traps and Snares

Introduction

Traps of various designs have been used since humankind learned to hunt. They form an important part of the arsenal of methods employed, worldwide, to control the so-called vermin species, to catch fur-bearing animals and to trap animals for food or the live animal trade. Although trap design has evolved in parallel in different parts of the world, the basic concepts and principles are universal: ensnaring, foot- or leg-hold devices, cages or nets.

Traps and snares may, and often do, injure the victim and in so doing may cause characteristic lesions that are valuable during investigations of illegal killings or other offences relating to trapping. Specific types of damage and, indeed, the absence of certain injuries can provide clues to the events preceding the death or release of the captured animal.

Spring traps

Spring traps have spring-loaded jaws that are released when pressure is applied to a trigger or plate in the centre of the trap (Fig. 11.1). Some of these traps, known as 'body grip' traps and 'humane spring traps', are designed to kill by closing on the body of small creatures such as rats, squirrels, stoats, weasels, mink and rabbits (Fig. 11.2).

Regulations vary around the world as to which traps may be used, and on their placement, to ensure that 'non-target' species (e.g. domestic cats) are not caught accidentally. The restrictions may, for example, require that traps are set in natural or artificial tunnels, that they are checked at specific periods (e.g. every 24 hours) and that any trapped animals are removed. The forensic veterinarian may be asked to determine whether the animal has been in the trap for longer than the maximum allowable period.

The jaws of the trap crush the chest and/or spine resulting in death. Animals caught in these traps show extensive internal injuries including fractured ribs, haemothorax, pulmonary laceration, ruptured liver and fracture of the thoracolumbar spine. The indentation marks of the jaws may be clearly seen across the body.

Use of spring traps for birds of prey

Body-grip spring traps designed for use on small animals may be misused to capture birds of prey. Baited traps are set in the open, in contravention of the regulations, and birds of prey trigger the trap by alighting on the trigger plate. The jaws close on the leg or legs of the bird, trapping, but not killing, the bird. Unable to extricate itself from the trap, the bird eventually dies from shock related to the severity of the leg injuries, dehydration and exhaustion. Any live bird in the trap may ultimately be killed by a blow from a stick or by dislocation of the neck (Fig. 11.3). It is, therefore, good practice to subject any 'found dead' bird of prey to a thorough post-mortem examination to determine the cause of death.

Leg lesions in birds caught in spring traps consist of abrasion and tearing of the skin, haemorrhage and fracture (frequently compound) of the tibiotarsal bone (Fig. 11.4). Some birds alight with one leg more extended than the other (e.g. buzzards). Those birds can suffer similar injuries to both legs but the lesions in the more extended leg are higher on that leg than those in the partially flexed leg.

In an attempt to mask or hide evidence that might indicate the bird has been caught in a spring trap, the jaws of the trap may be padded to lessen obvious injury to the legs. However, these padded jaws still exert considerable pressure and fracture of the tibiotarsal bone may occur. Additionally, the foot of the trapped leg may become considerably swollen and discoloured if the bird remains in the trap from some hours (Fig. 11.5).

Spring traps attached and set on the top of a fence-post in an open area with no other perching sites are referred to as 'pole' traps. These traps are unselective and trap one or both legs of the alighting bird. Once gripped around the leg(s) and unable to fly away, the exhausted bird may fall from the post to hang suspended by the trapped leg(s). In such cases, the legs may show the injuries described above and haemorrhage may be found in the muscles of the thigh and around the hip joint. Additionally, the head and neck may exhibit considerable congestion. Struggling may cause damage to feathers and bruising over bony prominences.

Leg- and foot-hold traps

These traps, like the body-grip traps, have a trigger and jaws to grip the prey. As the name suggests, leg-hold traps are designed to catch the leg or foot rather than the body. They are used for larger species such as wolves, foxes, coyotes, bobcats, racoons and feral cats.

Considerable efforts have been directed towards studying[1-6] and improving trap design to minimise injury, and some countries and states have taken steps to ban the use of the most injurious and cruel traps.

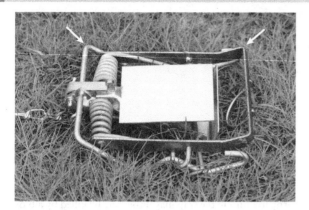

Fig. 11.1 – Spring trap in the 'set' position with the jaws (arrows) open. The flat metal plate in the centre is the trigger that 'springs' the jaws.

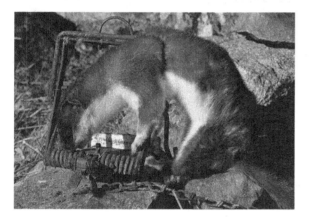

Fig. 11.2 – Weasel caught around the chest by a body-grip spring trap.

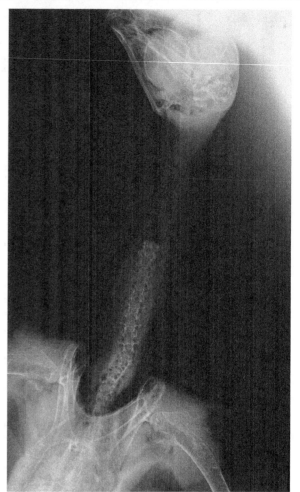

Fig. 11.3 – Goshawk. Radiography showing separation of cervical vertebrae from head following manual 'pulling' of the neck.

Soft tissue lesions include oedema (with or without haemorrhage) and laceration of skin and muscle (Fig. 11.6). Muscle injury may be accompanied by damage to tendons and ligaments or dislocation of elbow, hock and toe joints. Over-exertion, caused by attempts to escape from a protracted period of entrapment, can lead to degenerative changes in the muscles (exertional rhabdomyolysis).

Radiography is an essential part of the examination of animals when there is suspicion of trapping. Fractures may be found in the toes and foot or the long bones further up the limb. These fractures may be simple or compound (Fig. 11.7). Padded traps cause significantly less injury to the target species than steel-jawed traps, but may still result in serious injuries (e.g. limb fractures) to smaller non-target species.

Leg/foot-hold traps may result in amputations of the digits, foot or lower part of the limb (Fig. 11.8). Frostbite injuries and freezing of the limb may occur if the limb or foot is trapped for more than a few hours in ambient temperatures of −8°C or below.

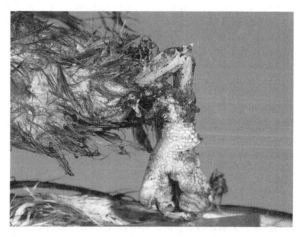

Fig. 11.4 – Buzzard. Compound fracture of the tibiotarsal bone caused by spring trap.

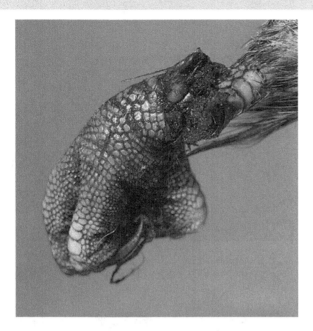

Fig. 11.5 – Buzzard. Fracture of the lower limb and marked swelling of the foot following prolonged entrapment in a spring trap.

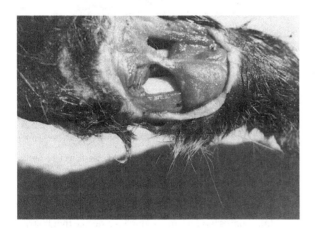

Fig. 11.6 – Racoon dog. Laceration of the skin and muscle of the forelimb caused by the teeth of a steel-jawed leg-hold trap.

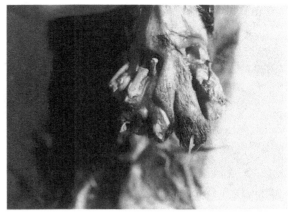

Fig. 11.7 – Racoon dog. Laceration and compound fractures of the digits caused by the teeth of a steel-jawed leg-hold trap.

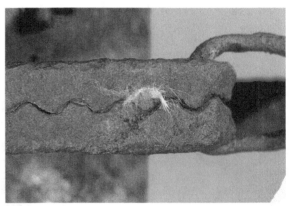

Fig. 11.8 – 'Gintrap'. This old fashioned illegal trap severed the lower hind limb of a rabbit. Note hair and blood on the closed jaws.

Mouth, teeth and jaw injuries are usually a consequence of biting at the trap in an attempt to escape (Fig. 11.9). Recent trap-related tooth injuries should be distinguished from pre-existing damage.

Foot-hold traps for beavers are normally set to catch the hind foot. If a forefoot is caught in error, this foot may be torn off during the subsequent struggle. Beaver traps are designed to drown the trapped animal, but several minutes of struggling may occur before the animal finally dies. The pathologist should look for signs of drowning and trauma related to the survival efforts.

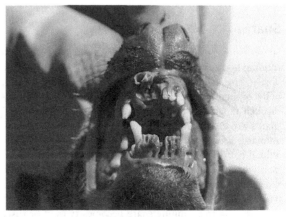

Fig. 11.9 – Racoon dog. Damage to teeth and jaws caused by frantic biting at leg-hold trap on forelimb.

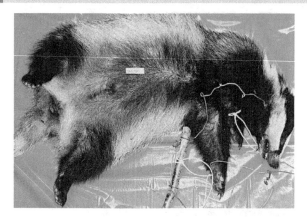

Fig. 11.10 – Badger. Trapped by wire snare encircling the neck.

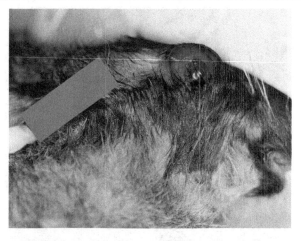

Fig. 11.12 – Hare. Compression of the jugular veins in the neck by a snare resulted in severe congestion of the head and haemorrhage into the right eye.

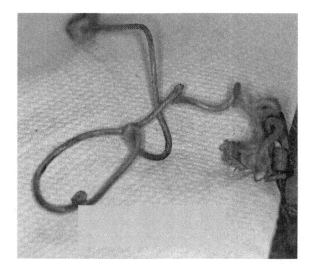

Fig. 11.11 – Twisted snare wire. Vigorous struggling by badgers, during attempts to escape, can result in marked twisting of the snare wire. Such a snare is no longer 'free-running' and tightens progressively.

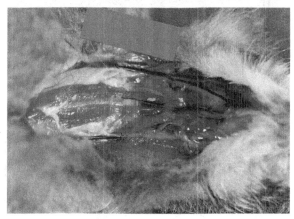

Fig. 11.13 – Hare (same animal as in Fig. 11.12). Dissection of the neck of the hare revealed the sharp contrast between the congested upper neck (to right of photograph) and the paler, normal tissue to the left.

Snares

Snares consist of a length of wire or cable, formed into a running noose, which is attached to a heavy or immovable object. The snare tightens when part of the animal (neck, body or limb) enters the snare but is too large to pass through it without dragging at the noose. 'Free-running' snares are designed to slacken when the pressure by the animal is released and, by doing so, continue to hold the animal but do not cause excessive tightening of the noose. 'Self-locking' snares do not slacken when the pressure on the noose is reduced and are banned in some countries because of their inherently cruel design. Unfortunately, if the wire of a free-running snare becomes twisted or rusty it can no longer slacken and, in effect, becomes self-locking (Figs 11.10 & 11.11).

Many snares have a 'stop', which is a device that restricts the extent to which the snare can tighten, thereby providing a degree of protection from over-tightening that might lead to strangulation of, say, the foot before the animal is released or killed by the trapper. This type of protection is of little value when a non-target species is caught in a snare designed for a smaller animal. In such a case, the noose of the snare strangulates (Figs 11.12 & 11.13) or cuts into the tissues before the restriction of the 'stop' comes into play (Fig. 11.14).

Badgers have comprehensive legal protection in some countries, yet illegal snaring is not uncommon. Badgers may die in snares as a result of:

- Injuries directly related to the snare wire
- Excessive struggling leading to trauma such as peritonitis following rupture of the intestines

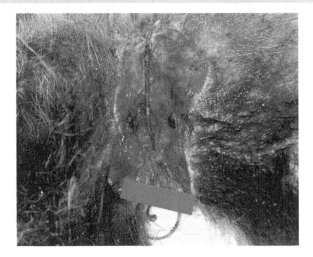

Fig. 11.14 – Badger. The snare encircling the chest cut through the skin, fat, muscle and eventually the sternum. The badger suffocated when air entered the chest and the lungs collapsed. He may have been in the snare for some days.

- Dehydration and starvation (if the snare is not visited for an extended period)
- Gunshot by the trapper.

The bodies of snared badgers are often buried to hide the evidence. Before discovery, these cadavers can suffer moderate to marked decomposition but this should not dissuade the forensic pathologist from conducting a detailed post-mortem examination.

If the badger is in the snare for several days, the snare wire may become embedded in the tissues and may remain attached to the buried cadaver. X-ray examination showing the wire *in situ* provides graphic evidence of the noose (Fig. 11.15). Soft tissue injuries in these cases may be obvious, consisting of a deep encircling wound marking where the noose cut into the neck or body before the animal died. Snared badgers are frequently shot, and radiography provides confirmation.

In other cases, the snare may have been removed before disposal of the cadaver and the skin may not be obviously marked. However, careful examination, from different angles, may detect indentations in the hair of the neck where the snare had tightened (Fig. 11.16). The underlying skin may show no obvious abrasion but reflection of the skin from the neck may reveal a pale line highlighting the compression of blood vessels, within the skin of the neck, by the snare wire (Fig. 11.17). Occasionally the hyoid is fractured. This may be found during the initial radiographic examination or when the structures of the throat and larynx are dissected. The larynx may be deeply congested and blood found in the windpipe. Haemorrhage may occur into the pleural cavity and the lungs are usually very congested and dark. Extensive pink froth in the windpipe and bronchi, and intra-alveolar haemorrhage and alveolar distension

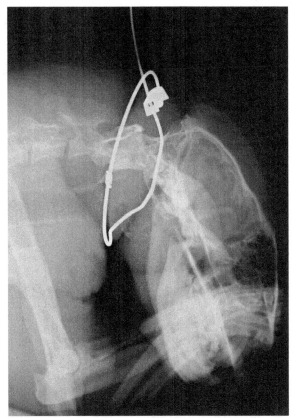

Fig. 11.15 – Radiograph of disinterred badger showing snare around neck.

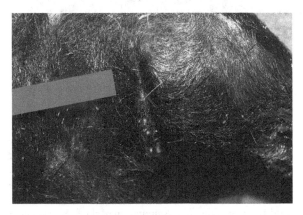

Fig. 11.16 – Badger. Groove on external surface of neck of a badger that had been snared, removed from the snare and buried.

(seen on microscopic examination) are consistent with death by strangulation.

Deer may also be caught in snares (Fig. 11.18). Depending on the type of snare, the noose may encircle the neck or the lower limb. Deer that survive for a period after being

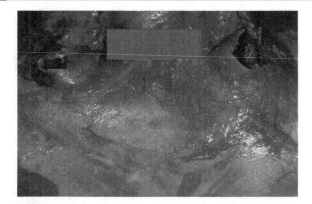

Fig. 11.17 – Badger. Blanched line on the inner surface of the skin of the neck showing line of compression where the snare encircled the neck. Death was by strangulation.

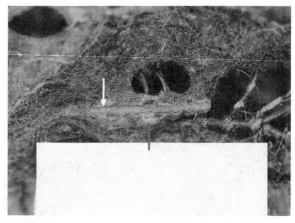

Fig. 11.19 – Squirrel. Desiccated body retrieved from cage trap. Note linear mark (white arrow) and surrounding rust stains (red arrow) indicating where the body rested on the cage floor for an extended period.

Cage traps

Cage traps are used for a wide range of mammals (e.g. rats, cats, foxes, squirrels, badgers) and some birds (e.g. crows and magpies).

Well designed and maintained cage traps limit injuries to mammals to relatively minor lesions such as abrasions arising from rubbing against the bars or mesh. However, a small percentage of animals may suffer more serious dental damage[7] through biting the bars or wire mesh.

A more serious problem is dereliction of duty on the part of the trapper by failure to inspect the trap at the required regular intervals, which may be once or twice in a 24-hour period. In severe cases, trapped animals may die from dehydration and starvation. Examination of the skeletalised remains covered by dried skin and hair may at first appear an unrewarding task. However, radiography may eliminate gunshot wounds as a cause of death and the presence of wire mesh markings on the coat of the undersurface of the animal may support other evidence pointing to long-term incarceration in the cage (Fig. 11.19). Should portions of internal organs be present then it may be appropriate to send these for toxicological analysis. As in many forensic examinations, estimation of the time of death may be of some importance (see Chapter 13: Estimation of time since death).

There are several different types and modifications of live cage traps for birds. Common designs include a 'ladder' or 'funnel' that allows birds to enter the trap (to retrieve food) by partially folding their wings and descending through an opening in the top. In order to escape, the birds must fly up to the hole in the roof but because of their extended wings they are unable to pass through the opening. Another common live cage trap is the Larsen trap, which has two compartments, one of which houses the 'call' bird that attracts others of the same species to enter the catching

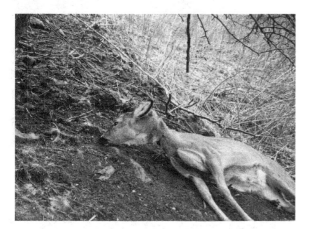

Fig. 11.18 – Roe deer caught by neck snare. Note constriction of neck, bareness of surrounding ground (caused by prolonged struggling) and clumps of hair on ground. Death was by strangulation. (By kind permission of the Scottish Society for the Prevention of Cruelty to Animals.)

caught may show severe skin wounds caused by the snare wire. Neck nooses result in death by strangulation, choking on regurgitated rumen contents or by hypovolaemic shock accompanied by acute renal failure. Leg/foot snares may cause local injury consisting of abrasion, tearing of the skin and swelling of the foot. Amputation of the foot may occur if the deer survives an extended period in the snare or if the deer escapes with the wire tightly fixed around the leg or foot. Exertional rhabdomyolysis with accompanying renal failure may supervene in leg-snared deer. Trappers may kill deer, found alive in snares, by shooting in the head or neck with a shotgun. However, post-mortem examination will detect snare injuries to the lower leg, and higher in the leg there may be muscle haemorrhage associated with struggling.

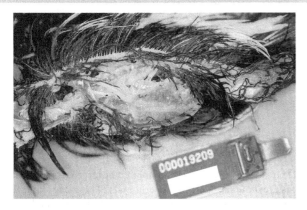

Fig. 11.20 – Magpie. Post-mortem predation of the pectoral region of a magpie that died from dehydration in a cage trap. Three other magpies in the cage survived.

chamber. Food, water, shelter and perches should be provided and the traps must be visited regularly to release or dispatch any trapped birds. Regulations governing the use of this type of trap, and the species that can be taken legally, vary from country to country.

Birds held for the recommended times in correctly maintained cage traps should not show significant injury. However, when the birds are held for extended periods, the tips of the primary feathers and the tail feathers may become dirty or abraded. If the cage floor is very dirty, marked faecal soiling may occur on the feet, wings, tail and feathers on the underside and around the vent. Birds left unattended in the traps without food and water may die and be predated upon by other trapped birds (Fig. 11.20).

Injuries can occur in poorly maintained traps when birds attempt to escape through rusty or broken wire mesh. These consist of skin punctures or tears, or damage to feathers.

Occasionally, trapped birds are deliberately and cruelly treated. When birds, within (or in the vicinity of) cages that conform to the recommended standards, are found to have fractured wings or legs there must be grave concern that the injuries have been caused deliberately.

References

1. Fleming PJS, Allen LR, Berghout MJ et al. The performance of wild-canid traps in Australia: efficiency, selectivity and trap-related injuries. Wildlife Res 1998; 25:237–338.

2. Kalmer JF, Richardson C, Gipson PS. Comparison of standard and modified Soft Catch® traps for capturing coyotes, bobcats, and raccoons. The Ninth Wildlife Damage Management Conference Proceedings, 5–8 October 2000, State College, PA; 2000.

3. Kreeger TJ, White PJ, Seal US, Tester JK. Pathological responses of red foxes to foothold traps. J Wildlife Manage 1990; 54:147–160.

4. Molster RL. Trapping and demographics of feral cats (*Felis catus*) in central New South Wales. Wildlife Res 2001; 28:631–636.

5. Onderka DK, Skinner DL, Todd AW. Injuries to coyotes and other species caused by four models of foothold devices. Wildlife Soc Bull 1990; 18:175–182.

6. Sahr DP, Knowlton FF. Evaluation of tranquilizer trap devices (TTDs) for foothold traps used to capture gray wolves. Wildlife Soc Bull 2000; 28:597–605.

7. Woodroffe R, Bourne FJ, Cox DR et al. Welfare of badgers (*Meles meles*) subjected to culling: patterns of trap-related injury. Anim Welfare 2005; 14:11–17.

Introduction

There are two immediate issues to be addressed when examining an animal with possible bite injuries. The first is to decide whether the lesions *are* the result of bites. The second is the differentiation of *dog* bite injury from that caused by other predators such as foxes, cats (large or small), ferrets, otters, badgers, mink, stoats, etc.

Some of the features that help decide which species may have inflicted the injuries are common sense. For example, the relative sizes of the predator and the victim are important. Thus, it would be extremely unlikely that a European otter would attack a Texel ram by biting it over the shoulder blades. Distribution of puncture marks may also give clues to the attacker. Cats commonly kill by biting the neck and head to immobilise the prey quickly and prevent struggling. This is particularly true if the victim is relatively large. Stoats show similar tactics when killing birds, chicks being wounded over the sternum and furculum (wishbone) whereas bigger birds are bitten on the head and neck.[1] Dogs, however, bite whatever they can.

Other useful clues to predator type include estimates of the size of the mouth, calculated by measuring the intercanine distance of 'bite pairs'. This is straightforward if the investigation requires a distinction to be made between a ferret and a Doberman pinscher. It is less easy if there is an overlap in jaw size, as occurs, for example, with a ferret to a young cat.[1]

The anatomy of the teeth and the biting process influence the marks left. The sharp canine teeth of the cat readily cause distinct puncture wounds, but the relatively blunt teeth of the dog do not penetrate skin so easily. Although foxes are often considered to have sharper pointed canine teeth than dogs, care should be taken in attempting to differentiate fox-bite marks from those of similarly sized dogs. Other clues (e.g. witness accounts, claw marks, footprints, and clear evidence of predation rather than attack) may be invaluable in assisting with decision-making in these cases.

Dog-bite injuries

From a veterinary perspective, forensic investigations of bite injuries are more commonly related to dog attack than biting by other animals.

Hares

Hares are usually caught and injured by large fast dogs such as greyhounds, Salukis or deerhounds. These dogs hunt by sight, catch up with the fleeing hare, and bite the body.

In a series of 53 hares examined by the Universities Federation for Animal Welfare (UFAW),[2] 79% suffered abdominal injury, 77% had chest injury and 74% damage to the hind limbs. Research commissioned by the Hunting with Dogs Inquiry in England showed somewhat similar results with 75% of hares with chest injuries, 41% with abdominal damage and 58% with significant bites to the hind limbs.[3]

Detailed examination in the authors' laboratories of seven hares, each killed on separate occasions by greyhounds or lurchers, revealed that the external appearance of these hares was highly misleading. Cursory examinations revealed only leakage of blood from the nostrils and irregular loss of hair from the hind limbs. *No punctures of the skin were present despite massive injury to the chest and abdomen.* From a forensic viewpoint, it is essential that thorough post-mortem examination is conducted and that reliance is not placed on the lack of obvious bite marks.

Chest injuries

Chest injuries consist of fractures of multiple ribs, irregular holes in the chest wall (Fig. 12.1) (often associated with the fractured ends of ribs), emphysema in the chest wall, puncture wounds and laceration of the lungs, haemothorax and, occasionally, puncture wounds to the heart. The sternum and the spinous processes of the thoracic vertebrae may be fractured during these attacks. These major thoracic injuries are accompanied by extensive subcutaneous and intramuscular haemorrhage over the chest walls, shoulder and back (Fig. 12.2).

Abdominal injuries

Abdominal injuries include severe subcutaneous haemorrhage, laceration of the abdominal wall, intra-abdominal haemorrhage, rupture of the liver, rupture of the diaphragm, perirenal haemorrhage, and puncture wounds to the stomach and intestines.

Other injuries

Subcutaneous and intramuscular haemorrhages are regular features in the hind limbs but fractures of the long bones

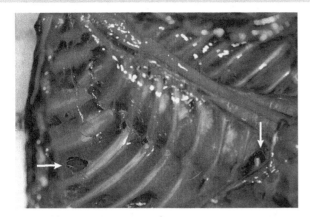

Fig. 12.1 – Hare. Extensive injury to chest caused by lurcher dog. Note multiple rib fractures and tears in chest wall (two tears are arrowed).

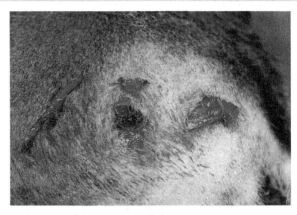

Fig. 12.3 – Roe deer. Dog bite wounds in skin over upper part of left hind limb and pelvis.

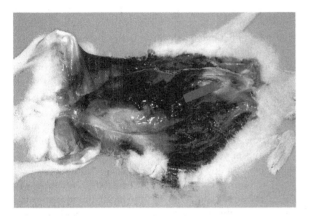

Fig. 12.2 – Hare. Extensive subcutaneous and intramuscular haemorrhage over chest and right side of abdomen caused by lurcher dog.

are uncommon. Other injuries include fractures of the scapula, fracture–dislocations of the lumbar or thoracic spine, and crush damage to the lumbar vertebrae and pelvis. Serious head injuries appear to be infrequent. Fracture or dislocation of the neck can occur during dog attack but are more commonly inflicted by the handler after picking up a non-fatally wounded hare.

Doubts have frequently been raised over the diagnosis of 'biting injury' in the absence of holes in the skin, not only in hares but also in other animals. From a lay viewpoint this is understandable. However, the forensic veterinarian should make it clear that puncture wounds in the skin are *not* an essential element of dog-bite injury. The same is true for badger bites of smaller creatures where fatal crush injuries to the chest are caused by single, well directed bites over the back and thorax.[4]

Differentiation of the injuries sustained by hares attacked by dogs from those arising in motor vehicle accidents relies on the same diagnostic pointers that are valuable in the investigation of the cause of injuries to dogs and cats (see Chapter 3: Non-accidental injury). The absence of oil and grease marks, abrasions, head injuries or long bone fractures, when combined with the pattern of the injuries described above, should leave little doubt as to the cause.

Deer

On catching up with a fleeing deer, a dog bites whatever it can. Consequently, severe injuries to the hindquarters of roe deer are typical of lurcher/greyhound attack. If more than one dog is involved, the second dog may also bite the hind end or, because the deer has been slowed by the initial attack, may go to the front of the deer and seize the throat.

In contrast to the situation in hares, where puncturing of the skin by dog bites is frequently absent, irregular tears and punctures in the skin over the posterior aspects of the hind limbs and the ischium are commonly found in deer subject to dog attack. These skin lesions, although obvious, may appear relatively minor (Fig. 12.3) and, as such, pose a danger for the unwary pathologist because they may belie the severity of the underlying lesions. The bites can cause extensive laceration of muscle (Fig. 12.4) and severe subcutaneous and intramuscular haemorrhage. Violent struggling as the deer attempts to escape may compound the injuries, resulting in extensive tearing of the adductor muscles of both hind limbs. Similar damage can occur over the lumbar region.

Dog attack to the throat of roe deer may leave the skin and hair virtually unmarked (Fig. 12.5). Suspicion of dog attack may not be raised until the skin of the neck is reflected to reveal soft tissue damage and haemorrhage on the ventral surface around the trachea, jugular grooves and related muscle bundles. Head injuries that include skin abrasions and punctures, subcutaneous bruising, and

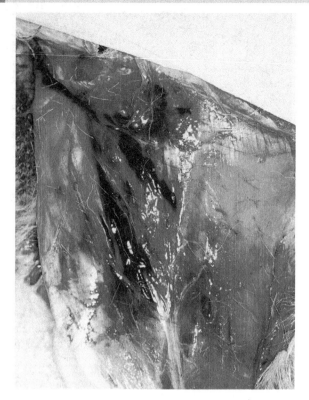

Fig. 12.4 – Roe deer. Laceration of muscle of left hind limb caused by dog bites. The overlying skin was intact.

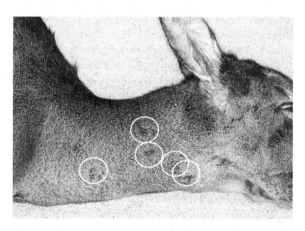

Fig. 12.5 – Roe deer. Minimal disturbance of coat (circles) and absence of puncture wounds in skin of neck following dog attack. Marked haemorrhage was present in underlying tissues.

haemorrhage around the eye or over the cranium may result from struggling rather than biting.

Bites to the legs or neck of deer may not be fatal and the dog owner may use a range of measures to kill the deer. Examples include dislocation of the neck, throat cuts and

shooting in the head with a low-velocity small-calibre bullet. Deer that escape despite being injured by the dogs may well die, after an extended period, as a result of the severe muscle injury combined with acute renal tubular necrosis induced by hypovolaemic shock.

Sheep

Sheep are vulnerable to attacks from dogs of various sizes – some large (e.g. German Shepherd), others smaller, such as collies, terrier types and spaniels. Study of livestock worrying in Australia indicates that two dogs are involved in the majority of attacks.[5]

The nature and site of the injuries is, to some extent, dependent on the size of the dog and the type of sheep. Large dogs are able to bite adults over the chest and lumbar region, and may cause fractures of lumbar and thoracic vertebral bodies, thoracic spinous processes, scapulae and humeri. Smaller dogs are less likely to fracture major bones but may inflict extensive injuries elsewhere.

Skin lesions range from no puncture wounds, to solitary puncture wounds, extensive tears or loss of portions of skin. Severe laceration and bruising, particularly of the head, throat region and hind limbs, are reported in sheep sent to the abattoir following dog worrying.[6] Over the head, puncture wounds in the skin may be present, and in lambs the skin injuries may be accompanied by skull fractures and punctures of the skull. The shaking and tearing elements of a dog attack may result in multiple injuries.

The biting process occurs in a dynamic situation with both the sheep and the dog moving. Consequently, it is seldom possible to identify a 'set' of teeth marks that corresponds to the size and shape of the mouth of a particular dog. Rather, individual holes or laceration may give an indication of the size of the dog by the depth of penetration of, say, a large canine tooth.

Birds

Dogs may gain access to poultry houses and game-bird pens, inflicting heavy losses. Alternatively they may enter a private garden and decimate the pet bantams. In all cases, great distress is caused to the birds and the owners. Occasionally, singleton wild birds are presented for examination with injuries that raise suspicion of dog-bite injuries. It is a generally accepted belief that cats (large and small) will bite the neck and head of birds, whereas dogs seize the body and wings. However, there is much variation, with cats biting small birds over the chest, and dogs inflicting wounds to the lower neck at the same time as biting the body. 'Soft-mouthed' breeds such as Labradors may pick up birds but inflict no physical injuries.

Comparison of injuries caused to domestic geese by a dog and by a large cat (suspected to be a European lynx) is informative (Fig. 12.6, Table 12.1) The difference in the *modus operandi* of the attacks is reflected in the injuries sustained by the geese.

The feathers frequently mask the severity of dog-bite injuries. Extensive subcutaneous haemorrhage may be present following crushing by even relatively small dogs. Careful plucking of the feathers (avoiding tearing the fragile skin) will reveal the extent of the bruising. Canine teeth do puncture avian skin but the holes often assume an elliptical shape rather than conforming to the outline of the tooth. Sometimes the hole in substantial muscle masses, e.g. the pectoral muscles, gives a better indication of the shape of the penetrating object. Internal injuries are often concentrated in the anterior part of the body cavity with haemorrhage being present over and within the lungs and in the air sacs.

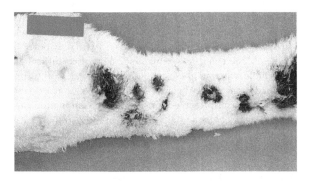

Fig. 12.6 – Domestic goose. Multiple bite wounds to the neck caused by a large cat (suspected to be a European lynx).

Bones in medium to small birds are generally of light construction and fracture readily. Fractures of the ribs, breastbone, spine and long bones of the wings are common. Gunshot wounds also fracture these bones and radiography is an essential tool in the investigation of the injuries.

Foxes

There are three major scenarios in which dogs inflict bites to foxes:

1. The fox is caught above ground by a pack of foxhounds.
2. The fox is set upon above ground by a lurcher, or similar type of dog, accompanied by one or more terriers.
3. The fox is injured underground by a terrier.

Foxhound pack

The cadavers of these foxes are extensively damaged by multiple bites, some ante mortem, others post mortem.[7] Attempts should be made at post-mortem examination, by reference to haemorrhage and soft tissue bruising, to separate the ante-mortem injuries from those inflicted after death as the pack tears at the cadaver.

Fatal injuries are concentrated in the chest and abdomen, and consist of crushing of the chest wall, multiple fractures of ribs, fractures of thoracic and/or lumbar spine, severe laceration of the lungs, rupture of the diaphragm, rupture of the abdominal wall and destruction of the abdominal organs. Fractures of the limbs and pelvis are also features

Table 12.1 Comparison of dog and large cat attacks on domestic geese

	Dog attack	Large cat attack
Weight of goose	4.3 kg	5.9 kg
Neck	Not injured	Multiple bites (12 on left, 10 on right) Massive haemorrhage Spinal cord severed
Back	Four puncture wounds in skin, 2–6 mm in diameter Subcutaneous haemorrhage Laceration of muscles 4–30 mm in length	Not injured
Chest	Four puncture wounds on right side accompanied by extensive haemorrhage, laceration of muscles and fracture of ribs Extensive haemorrhage within chest cavity Laceration of right lung	Five puncture wounds of right ventral chest (claw marks) Five puncture wounds and slit wounds in pectoral muscles deep to skin wounds Three fractured ribs on left side Liver ruptured
Cause of death	Crushing of chest Haemorrhage into chest Laceration of lung	Neck trauma with severance of spinal cord

of these attacks. Serious head and neck injuries are not major features of this type of attack.

Lurchers

Again the fatal injuries are concentrated in the chest and back areas. Fractures of the spinous processes of the thoracic vertebrae, fractured ribs, puncturing of the chest wall, laceration of the lungs, extensive haemorrhage over chest and abdominal walls, groin and hind limbs are significant features. Bite wounds may also be found in muscles of the hind and forelimbs. Bruising in the neck may result from biting or shaking.

Terriers

The terrier's job is to locate and keep the fox in the hole. Digging then exposes the fox, and the terrier is removed. If the fox is still alive, it is shot.

Terrier attack is not necessarily fatal and the wounds to the fox may be concentrated at the front of the fox. Thus, there may be multiple bite wounds to the face, top of head, forelimbs and lower neck.

Dogs and cats

Dog-bite wounds often consist of a mixture of crushing and irregular tearing injuries that are created as one canine tooth 'serves as an anchorage, while the other teeth cut into the flesh causing stretch lacerations in the process of biting, shaking and tearing' (De Munnynck & Van de Voorde 2002, p 298)[8]. Relatively minor skin lesions may mask severe laceration and avulsion of underlying muscle, damage to vasculature and, possibly, internal organs.[9–11] Limb bones, skull and vertebrae may be fractured, and the chest or abdominal wall breached.

The reported distribution of these injuries in dogs varies, with limb, head and neck, thorax and abdomen, and perineum (in descending order of frequency) being noted in North America,[10] whereas the thorax, extremities, limb and tail, and head and neck are the common sites in Israel.[11] These differences may be a reflection of the different sizes of dogs in the populations studied, as small dogs sustain the most thoracic injuries whereas larger dogs have the highest prevalence of head wounds.[11] Similarly, injuries to multiple body regions are more common in small dogs compared with larger breeds.

Less detailed information is available on dog-bite injuries to cats, but damage to the back, thorax and abdomen appears to be most prevalent.

Children

Veterinarians may be asked to examine dogs suspected of involvement in attacks on children. The veterinary investigations should include careful collection of evidence such as blood, hairs and fibres from the coat and mouth, and the veterinary history of the dog should be studied for evidence of previous behavioural problems or for recent administration of veterinary medicines. Urine analysis for stimulating substances can be valuable and provides background information on the domestic situation. If the suspect dog is euthanased, a full post-mortem examination should be undertaken with a view to recording any pathological conditions that might have affected behaviour. The oral and gastric contents should be submitted to a (human) forensic science laboratory to be examined for traces of human blood or tissue or clothing.

Neonatal and post-mortem predation

From time to time the question arises as to whether a calf, or lamb, died and was subsequently the target of predation or whether the newborn was attacked around the time of parturition. Many of these cadavers are moderately autolysed before being presented for examination. In others, all internal organs are missing with only portions of head, chest and legs remaining. It is often difficult to determine whether these animals were dead at the time of predation. Nevertheless, if the cadaver is reasonably intact and well preserved, post-mortem examination may detect clear evidence that the animal was stillborn (e.g. uninflated lungs) or suffered from a life-threatening disease process.

Although there are reports of predators (e.g. jackals) attacking the face and removing the tongue from calves during prolonged parturition,[12] it is more common that weakly neonatal animals become comatose and die through hypothermia and hypoglycaemia before being the subject of predation. These cadavers may show gnaw marks on long bones or evidence of chewing of fractured rib ends. Such signs point to innocent predation of carrion rather than some savage attack on a defenceless creature.

References

1. Lyver PO'B. Identifying mammalian predators from bite marks: a tool for focusing wildlife protection. Mammal Rev 2000; 30:31–44.

2. Universities Federation for Animal Welfare. Research and investigations, hares. Annual Report 1979:7–9.

3. Report of the Committee of Enquiry into Hunting with Dogs in England and Wales. Final research reports: Hare postmortems. Accompanying CD to CM 4763. Crown copyright 2000.

4. Michener GR, Iwaniuk AN. Killing technique of North American badgers preying on Richardson's ground squirrels. Can J Zool 2001; 79:2109–2113.

5. Jennens G. Dog attacks on livestock. Urban Animal Management Conference Proceedings, Perth, Australia, 1998. Online Available: http://pandora-test.nla.gov.au/parchive/2001/Z2001-Feb-5/www.farmwide.com.au/nff/vetasscn/confer/uam/proc98/jennens.htm 16 Oct 2007.

6. Thornton H, Gracey JF. Textbook of meat hygiene, 6th edn. London: Baillière Tindall; 1974.

7.   Report of the Committee of Enquiry into Hunting with Dogs in England and Wales. Final research reports: Fox postmortems. Accompanying CD to CM 4763. Crown copyright 2000.

8.   De Munnynck K, Van de Voorde W. Forensic approach to fatal dog attacks: a case report and literature review. Int J Legal Med 2002; 116:295–300.

9.   Cowel AK, Penwick RC. Dog bite wounds: a study of 93 cases. Compendium on Continuing Education for the Practicing Veterinarian 1989; 11:313–320.

10. Holt DE, Griffin G. Bite wounds in dogs and cats. Vet Clin North Am Small Anim Pract 2000; 30:669–679.

11. Shamir MH, Leisner S, Klement E et al. Dog bite wounds in dogs and cats. J Vet Med [Ser A] 2002; 49:107–112.

12. Yom-Tov Y, Ashkenazi S. Cattle predation by the golden jackal in the Golan Heights, Israel. Biol Conserv 1995; 73:19–22.

13 | Estimation of Time since Death

Introduction

The 'time since death', or post-mortem interval, is the time that has elapsed between the death of an animal and the discovery of the body. Establishment of this interval aids investigation of the circumstances surrounding the death by narrowing the 'window of time' during which the death may have occurred. In so doing, specific people or events may be excluded, or included, in the investigations that follow.

In human forensic medicine, study of the post-mortem interval has been one of the most popular topics of research.[1] However, bedevilled as it is by the sheer variety of species involved, estimation of the post-mortem interval is much less developed in veterinary medicine. Indeed, there is a marked paucity of published information. Some attempts have been made with certain species of North American deer and other wildlife.[2-7] A more recent study that involved recording of post-mortem rectal temperatures and macroscopic and microscopic changes in a limited number of Beagles provides a practical approach to the development of a standardised method for the estimation of the time since death in dogs.[8] However, this study was restricted to specific environmental conditions (10.9–16.8°C) and dogs weighing between 8.5 and 15 kg.

The veterinarian may become involved in widely differing incidents, including out-of-season shooting of game animals, poaching, death of livestock during transport, and cases of neglect or deliberate injury of companion animals. Additionally, estimation of the time since death may also be important when two or more animals are found at a single location. In such cases the veterinarian needs to determine, if possible, whether the deaths occurred as a result of a single event or as part of an ongoing, lengthier process. Determination of the time of death may have relevance to cases where the alleged offences are related to statutory time limits, e.g. checking of traps within defined periods, or disposal of carcasses.

The focus of an inquiry or intended prosecution will be influenced by the estimate of the post-mortem interval. This places a considerable responsibility on the veterinarian. If the estimate is inaccurate to a major degree, then time will be wasted on unproductive investigations and suspects may be charged unjustly.

In most cases it is impossible to establish the *precise* time of death. Consequently, the estimated time is best presented as a range based on minimum and maximum times.

The current state of knowledge should allow the experienced pathologist, in the normal course of events, to estimate the post-mortem period in blocks of time, such as less than 24 hours, 1–3 days, 3–7 days, 7–21 days, weeks, months or years. However, it is important that all parties are aware of the limited information available and that the Courts are not inadvertently persuaded that 'time since death' estimates are based on a firm and substantial data base.

Box 13.1

Methods for estimation of the post-mortem interval

Temperature-based methods
Rigor mortis
Electrical stimulation
Eye changes
Decomposition
    a) gross pathology
    b) histopathology
Entomology
Environmental and associated evidence

Temperature-based methods

Countless crime novels and television murder dramas have reinforced the popular misconception that a single simple measurement of rectal temperature provides a reliable estimate of the post-mortem interval. In reality, cooling of the body is affected by many factors including insulation, ambient temperature, movement of air and immersion in water. Consequently, much investigation has been devoted to the effects of these variables on the cooling curve of the human cadaver. The results of this research have been incorporated into nomograms that, when used in conjunction with accurate measurement of core body temperature, provide reasonably tight maximum and minimum time limits.[9]

Similar nomograms have yet to be developed for domestic and free-living animals. As mentioned in the introduction to this chapter, some effort has been expended in attempting to create guidelines for cooling rates in some species of North American deer. Some of these methods are solely temperature based, whereas others combine temperature measurements and other changes such as pupil diameter or aqueous humour biochemistry.

Because many deer are field-dressed (i.e. the abdominal cavity is opened and the stomach and intestines are removed) shortly after death, rectal temperatures are inappropriate. In these cases, temperature measurement is made in the muscles of the thigh and intranasally. The rectum and cloaca are the usual sites for temperature recording in smaller mammals and birds.

Despite data being available on body surface area and body mass for different species, considerable care needs to be exercised during interpretation of post-mortem temperatures in wildlife. This caution is based on the inherent uncertainties that are commonplace in wildlife investigations. For example, there will be a lack of reliable information on ante-mortem body temperature, which may have been raised by physical exertion before death. Similarly, the actual influence of post-mortem handling procedures, including skinning, transportation on the roof of a vehicle or transportation within a closed vehicle with animals piled one on another, is as yet incompletely investigated.

On the domestic animal front, the cooling rates of carcasses of farm livestock slaughtered in abattoirs are well researched. However, there are no published accounts of studies on estimation of the post-mortem interval of similar animals found dead, but intact, in a farmyard or field.

The study by Erlandsson & Munro[8] on beagles showed that over the first 10 hours after death rectal temperature could be helpful in establishing the approximate time of death within intervals, or time bands, of 2 hours. Further, under the conditions of the study (dogs lying undisturbed in cool dry air), body temperature declined to ambient temperature by 24–48 hours after death. Additional data are required on the effects on the cooling curve of higher ambient temperatures, different body weights, moving air, coverings and immersion in water.

Rigor mortis

Fully developed rigor mortis is an easily identifiable and reliable indicator that death has occurred. The time of onset is variable but it is usually considered to appear between 1 and 6 hours (average 2–4 hours) after death. Depending on the circumstances, rigor mortis may last for a few hours to several days.

The muscles of the face and neck are often the first to be affected and the rigidity spreads backwards over the trunk and limbs. Relaxation of the muscles occurs in roughly the same order. Contraction of the heart is an early and forceful change. In the healthy, non-hypoxic animal the left ventricle expels virtually all its contents of blood during this process, whilst contracture of the right ventricle is less intense, leaving a small quantity of clotted blood in this chamber.

The development and resolution of rigor mortis is complex, the rate of onset being greatly influenced by the glycogen content of muscle, the pH of muscle and the temperature. Adenosine triphosphate (ATP) is a necessary component in the relaxation of the myosin filaments of normal muscle. *Rigor mortis* commences when the rate of re-synthesis of ATP is less than its degradation. In the early hours after clinical death, muscle glycogen fuels the cycle of hydrolysis and re-synthesis of ATP. Consequently, ante-mortem events that reduce glycogen stores (e.g. hunting) can result in the rapid onset of rigor mortis. In contrast, 9–12 hours may elapse after slaughter of well fed, well rested cattle before the onset of rigor mortis.

Body temperature also affects the rapidity of onset. The most dramatic example is the onset of rigidity within minutes in cases of malignant hyperthermia.[10,11] Following fatal hyperthermia of dogs in vehicles, less than 1 hour may pass before rigor mortis is recognisable and it may spread rapidly throughout the muscle groups. Raised body temperature as a consequence of severe exercise may also significantly shorten the time before rigor mortis develops.

However, the effects of increased body temperature are not always so clearcut and the presence of systemic disease must be considered. Whilst pyrexia caused by acute fatal infectious disease may result in rapid onset of rigor mortis, fevered animals with high muscle pH may show delayed rigor mortis or may not develop rigidity at any stage.

In general, high environmental temperature will accelerate the onset, whereas low ambient temperatures have the opposite effect. The duration of rigidity is extended in dry cold conditions. Although the details of the relaxation process are not clear, it is generally accepted that the dissolution of rigidity is associated with early decomposition or denaturisation of muscle.

For the veterinarian, a further complication is the, as yet, largely undocumented variation in the times of onset and disappearance of rigidity that may exist among species and ages of the broad spectrum of animals presented for examination. As a result of these variables, it is prudent to consider rigor mortis as providing only a rough guide to the post-mortem interval.

Electrical stimulation of skeletal muscles

Post-mortem electrical excitability of skeletal muscles of human cadavers has been examined in some detail.[12] Some attention has been paid to the application of this technique in the estimation of the time since death in wildlife. In deer, various sites for the electrodes have been used including eye, muzzle, ear, forelimb above elbow, along the back ventral to the thoracic vertebrae, tail, and inner thigh. In ducks, a detectable reaction in the wing suggests that the bird died less than 1 hour before testing, whereas in the goose a response may be recognised for up to 2 hours.[6]

A major drawback of current procedures, as they are applied to wildlife, is the reliance on subjective grading, by the operator, of muscular contraction. Additional research would appear to be required on objective methods of measurement of the force of muscle contraction and the shape of the recorded graphs at different times post mortem.

Decomposition

General

The study by James & Knight[13] showed that experienced human pathologists tend to under estimate the time since death. A similar situation may exist in veterinary pathology.

Following clinical death with cessation of blood circulation and respiration, the process of post-mortem decomposition of the body begins. Some tissues decompose faster than others, the breakdown of the body being driven, partly, by the release of enzymes and autolysis and, partly, by microbial action and colonisation by scavengers. This is an uneven process, possibly accelerated in one part of the body by external factors (warmth, oxygen, bacteria) but retarded in another by lower temperatures or dryness. Natural disease may also play a role in altering the expected rate of change. These processes are well described in standard veterinary pathology texts.[14,15]

Green discoloration of the ventral abdomen can be obvious in dogs within 24 hours of death. This colour usually strengthens over the succeeding days and the affected area enlarges. The colour develops because of post-mortem activity of micro-organisms in the intestines. Consequently, severely malnourished and dehydrated dogs and cats with virtually no intestinal contents show lesser colour change. (These malnourished animals are also usually less malodorous than well fed ones. Two main reasons for the reduced odour are more rapid cooling of the thin animal and the reduced bacterial activity in the intestines.) Colour changes are equally apparent in the abdominal organs. The kidneys, for example, may show rapid development of dark discoloration of the caudal poles where they lie adjacent to a well filled colon (see Fig. 6.24).

Caution is required when interpreting decomposition in ruminants, particularly in warm weather. Changes can be surprisingly rapid. The abdomen of sheep, cattle and deer that had access to plentiful, lush grazing before death may become bloated and discoloured within hours. The kidneys and liver may become soft and discoloured at the same time. Discoloration of the liver is frequently uneven as a result of post-mortem bacterial invasion along the portal vessels to the central veins and out into the surrounding sinusoids. The resulting mottled appearance has contributed to many misdiagnoses, by the unwary, of 'hepatopathy'.

From time to time gastric rupture is encountered in decomposing canine cadavers. The question that must be addressed is whether the rupture was causally related to the death or whether it is a post-mortem event. There seems little doubt that post-mortem gastric rupture with subsequent leakage of gastric contents into the peritoneal cavity

can occur in dogs. The affected animal is usually fairly decomposed but with the abdominal wall intact. The abdomen may be distended by gas within the peritoneal cavity and this gas escapes on first incision of the wall. Differentiation from ante-mortem gastric rupture rests on the absence of (1) evidence of gastric torsion, (2) evidence of trauma to the anterior abdomen, (3) ante-mortem lesions in the gastric wall and (4) inflammatory changes in the peritoneal surfaces.

The diaphragm can present a significant barrier to the spread of post-mortem invaders. Decomposition may be obvious in the abdominal organs but the lungs and heart may remain relatively fresh for some days. Erlandsson & Munro[8] noted blood-stained fluid in the thoracic cavity 7 days after death, but not at 3 days. Similar fluid was recorded in the pericardial sacs of dogs necropsied 23 days post mortem, but was absent at 7 days.

Freezing artefacts

Cadavers that have been chilled or frozen before necropsy frequently demonstrate generalised pink discoloration of the mucous membranes of the mouth, of the subcutaneous tissues, the muscles, the spinal cord, the serosal surface of the intestines and abdominal wall, and the tracheal mucosa. This colour should be differentiated from active and passive congestion, hypostasis and intoxication by carbon monoxide or cyanide.

Freezing undoubtedly has a detrimental effect on cell and tissue integrity. The extent of the damage influences decisions on collection of tissues for histopathology. The central nervous system is frequently rendered unsuitable for microscopy following freezing. Many artefacts can develop in parenchymatous organs such as the liver, but major lesions may remain recognisable. Muscle and dense fibrous tissue may show relatively little change.

Small quantities of watery, pink fluid regularly collect in the serous cavities after freezing and thawing. In most cases there should be little difficulty in differentiating this fluid from ante-mortem haemorrhage.

Burial and immersion

Specific events such as burial or immersion may materially affect the rate of decomposition. In general, burial in earth retards decomposition by ensuring a lower ambient temperature (except in winter), by exclusion of oxygen and by protection from scavengers (maggots, beetles, birds and mammals). Animals that are partially decomposed before burial will putrefy in the grave more rapidly than those buried soon after death. Deep burials may keep the body cooler than if placed in a shallow grave but, in either case, careful examination of an exhumed body may prove very worthwhile. Some cadavers may be remarkably well preserved and provide vital information on soft tissue damage. Bruising becomes less clear as decomposition advances, and

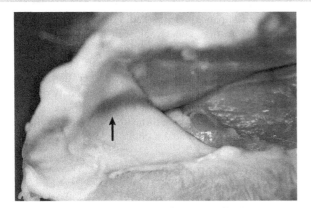

Fig. 13.1 – Kitten. Subcutaneous haemoglobin staining (arrow) arising from post-mortem diapedesis in a kitten that had been frozen 24 hours after death and thawed 7 days later.

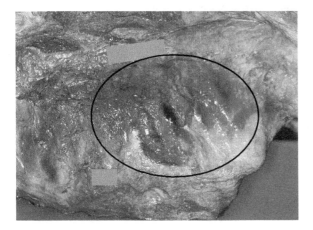

Fig. 13.2 – Dog. Extensive bruising (circled) over the left chest wall remains recognisable in an adult dog who had been buried for several weeks during warm weather.

haemoglobin staining arising from post-mortem diapedesis can, at first sight, mimic bruising (Fig. 13.1), but extensive bruising may remain clearly recognisable weeks or months after the body was interred (Fig. 13.2). Other exhumed bodies consist of little more that skeletalised remains and fragments of skin. However, even these may reveal unexpected bony fractures (recent or healed) or evidence of shooting.

Immersion in water generally slows the rate of putrefaction when compared to that seen a similar body left in the air. In veterinary forensic practice, dogs and cats that are deliberately drowned may be weighted down and are not discovered for an extended period after submersion. Despite the retarding effect of immersion in cold water, these bodies are frequently in an advanced state of decomposition when retrieved. The hair and epidermis are readily detached in places, leaving a slippery fawn–white covering of dermis and subcutaneous tissue. Marks caused by ligatures, used to bind legs or to attach weights to the neck, may be obvious

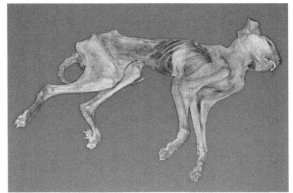

Fig. 13.3 – Mummified body of a cat found behind a partition in the inner wall of a building.

even if the ligatures have been removed before the cadaver is presented for post-mortem examination. Unusual marks, sometimes mimicking minor stab wounds of the skin, can be seen on seals and other sea mammals found on the seashore. These are post-mortem injuries caused by scavenging crustaceans.

Mummification

Accounts of individual mummified cats being found in basement rooms and cellars, where they may have lain for extended periods of time, appear from time to time. Few of these have any sinister connotations and are tragic accidents. Less commonly, dogs or other creatures are found dead in cupboards or elsewhere in houses. The circumstances surrounding this type of death merit investigation.

During the process of mummification the body becomes progressively dehydrated and the normal putrefactive decomposition is inhibited. It occurs most readily in a current of dry warm air. Although dryness is clearly necessary, exactly how warm the atmosphere needs to be is less certain. For example, companion animals abandoned in relatively cold, unoccupied houses in which one or more windows are open may become mummified. In these circumstances, as with any trapped animal, lack of availability of drinking water may be a crucial factor influencing development of mummification.

Small animals dry out more readily than larger ones. Mummification may involve the whole body or may be better developed in some parts than others. Depending on circumstances, mummification and other post-mortem changes such as adipocere formation or the usual liquefactive process may coexist in the same body.

Decomposition and post-mortem scavenging can proceed in tandem, resulting in a desiccated skeleton covered by dried skin and hair, but with only limited muscle tissue and no internal organs.

The skeleton may be tightly enveloped in virtually hairless, brown, hard skin that outlines the ribs (Fig. 13.3) and

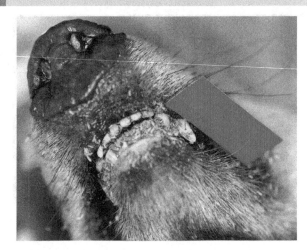

Fig. 13.4 – Badger. Numerous maggots in mouth and around teeth. Maggots were also present in the ears and on the skin of the axillae and abdomen.

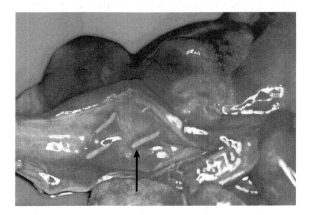

Fig. 13.5 – Kitten. Drowned and left outside in cool weather for 2 weeks in a cardboard box. Maggots in the oesophagus (arrow).

causes the lips to form a sinister grin. However, much of the hair may remain, giving the cadaver a relatively normal appearance when first sighted.

Anecdotal evidence suggests that partial mummification of dogs can occur in a few weeks. The process of complete mummification probably extends over many months.

Adipocere formation

Adipocere '*is caused by hydrolysis and hydrogenation of adipose tissue, leading to the formation of a greasy or waxy substance if of recent origin*' (Saukko & Knight 2004, p 70)[16]. It is off-white in colour but can become stained with haemoglobin and other products of the putrefactive process. As time passes it may become drier, brittle and chalk-like. Adipocere is remarkably stable; it may last for many years and may preserve the shape of the body and organs.

There is a paucity of information on the circumstances in veterinary work in which adipocere is found. Moist conditions aid the formation of adipocere and it might be expected to develop regularly in animals buried in wet graves. The lack of such accounts of adipocere may, merely, be a reflection of the low numbers of animals that are exhumed and examined. Based on the experience with human remains, adipocere formation should, typically, be visible to the eye around 3 months.[16]

Forensic entomology

Forensic entomology is a specialised area of investigation; reference to guidance notes[17] on collection and preservation of specimens is essential. Incorrect storage, e.g. immersion of live maggots in ethanol, may considerably reduce the value of the investigation and may lead to errors in estimation of larval age based on size.

Although blowfly larvae are the most important specimens for use in forensic entomology, other insects should also be collected, particularly if the cadaver is more than 10 days old.

Maggots are commonly found in and around the body orifices (Fig. 13.4), in wounds, on the skin of the head, between the foreleg and chest (axilla), over abdomen and on snares encircling the neck. Maggots also invade the body and may be found in the windpipe, gullet (Fig. 13.5) and body cavities. Green-bottles (*Lucilia*) and blue-bottles (*Calliphora*) migrate from the body once they have completed feeding, and search of the surrounding ground or carpets and furniture for puparia might detect a first wave of blowflies that would otherwise have been missed.

References

1. Knight B. The evolution of methods for estimation of the time of death from body temperature. Forensic Sci Int 1988; 36:47–55.
2. Woolf A, Roseberry JL, Will J. Estimating time of death of deer in Illinois. Wildlife Soc Bull 1982; 11:47–51.
3. Pex JO, Meneely KD, Andrews FC. Time of death estimation in blacktail deer by temperature and aqueous humour. J Forensic Sci 1983; 28:594–600.
4. Kienzler JM, Dahn PF, Fuller WA et al. Temperature based estimation for the time of death in white tailed deer. Biometrics 1984; 40:849–854.
5. Cox RJ, Mitchell SL, Epinoza EO. CompuTOD, A computer program to estimate time of death of deer. J Forensic Sci 1994; 39:1287–1299.
6. Adrian WJ. Wildlife forensic field manual, 2nd edn. Fort Collins, CO: Association of Midwest Fish and Game Law Enforcement Officers; 1996.
7. Hadley BM, Robbins LW, Beffa DA. Estimating the time of death of deer in Missouri: a comparison of three indicators. J Forensic Sci 1999; 44:1124–1130.
8. Erlandsson M, Munro R. Estimation of the post mortem interval in Beagle dogs. Science & Justice 2007; 47:150–154.
9. Henssge C. Temperature based methods II. In: Knight B, ed. The estimation of the time since death in the early post mortem period, 2nd edn. London: Arnold, 2002:43–102.

10. Hopkins PH, Ellis FR. Hyperthermic and hypermetabolic disorders: exertional heat-stroke, malignant hyperthermia and related syndromes. Cambridge: Cambridge University Press; 1996.

11. Williams DC, Brosman RJ, Aleman MR et al. Suspected malignant hyperthermia in a horse anaesthetized with halothane. Vet Anaesth Analg 2002; 29:91.

12. Madea B. Post mortem electrical excitability of skeletal muscle in case work. In: Knight B, ed. Estimation of the time since death in the early post mortem period, 2nd edn. London: Arnold; 2002:164–206.

13. James WRL, Knight BH. Errors in estimating time since death. Med Sci Law 1965; 5:111–116.

14. Jones TC, Hunt RD, King NW. Veterinary pathology, 6th edn. Baltimore: Williams & Wilkins; 1997.

15. Myers RK, McGavin MD. Cellular and tissue responses to injury. In: McGavin MD, Zachary JF, eds. Pathologic basis of veterinary disease, 4th edn. Edinburgh: Mosby Elsevier; 2007:25–28.

16. Saukko P, Knight B. Pathophysiology of death. In: Knight's forensic pathology, 3rd edn. London: Arnold; 2004:52–97.

17. Hall MJR. Collecting and preserving entomological material for forensic study. London: Department of Entomology, Natural History Museum; 2006.

14 | Sexual Abuse of Animals

Introduction

For thousands of years, the use of animals for sexual purposes has been recorded in many societies around the world.[1,2] Such activity has by no means always been tolerated; indeed, it has invariably been condemned for reasons that were often religious or moral in origin,[1,2] but also because some people are repelled by the very thought of interest in sexual activity with animals and find the subject abhorrent.[2,3] It is also a fact that embarrassment about the practice affects many people, from all walks of life (including some veterinarians), thus clouding judgement, making rational discussion difficult, and may even be a contributory factor to the paucity of information in English-language veterinary literature on injuries associated with the abuse.

Terminology

Most people are familiar with the term *bestiality*, the precise meaning of which has varied in the past but which currently is understood to mean sexual activity between a person and an animal. Unfortunately, the word bestiality, and its modern synonym *zoophilia*, both focus on the *person* involved, and as a result any harm that may be suffered by the animal is simply not considered. The term 'animal sexual abuse', which has developed from the now familiar term 'child sexual abuse', is preferable and more precise.[4,5]

What classifies the abuse as sexual?

In essence, it is the fact that the actions centre on the sexual organs, or the anus and rectum (and the cloaca in birds), that distinguishes this type of abuse as sexual in nature (Fig. 14.1).

Common sense dictates that whether an animal is physically harmed depends on the actual type of sexual contact and also the size of the animal. It should be realised that certain people who have very strong emotional attachments to their animals do exist, and that these attachments may take on a physical expression.[1,3] These particular owners are insistent that they would not knowingly physically harm their animals. On the other hand, there are people who are totally uncaring of the physical harm that they cause. Some of this physical harm can be extreme.

Veterinarians need to be aware of the existence of the sexual abuse of animals because their particular expertise will be called upon when injury occurs. However, they should focus on harm caused to the animals and avoid discussion of the reasons *why* the animals have been sexually abused.

Species and sex of animals used

It is a mistake to assume that the sexual activity consists solely of vaginal penile penetration of a farmyard animal by a man. The range of animals (and birds) used by humans for sexual purposes is extensive, and involves a wide variety of activities with both male and female animals by men and women, although women who take part appear to be fewer in number. Some activities may, on the face of it, seem harmless, but some result in severe physical harm and may even cause death. Reports generally appear in literature that is not readily available to (English speaking) veterinarians, and it is quite possible to remain unaware that these activities exist. It is also possible to be unaware of their important wider social aspects, such as the connection between sexual abuse of animals and the sexual abuse of children.[6,7] However, it is a fact that information is widely available on the internet. For example, information can be found on how to 'groom' animals (both males and females) for sexual activities, with additional advice as to appropriate size, so that the animal is not physically harmed.

Injuries

The sexual contacts employed include vaginal or anal penile penetration, penetration of the vagina or anus/rectum by an object (a stick or broom handle, for example) and wounds inflicted on, in, or around the genitalia. Depending on the type of sexual act carried out, and the size of the animal, damage can range from no injury to severe injuries. Fatalities can occur.

Only veterinarians have the skills to investigate the injuries associated with sexual abuse, but there is a remarkable paucity of information in English-language veterinary literature. For example, sexual abuse does not appear to be included in the differential diagnosis of vaginal lesions in veterinary obstetrics and gynaecology textbooks, nor has it been considered in texts describing lesions of the male genitalia and the anus and rectum of either sex. However, Reichert, describing a series of cases in cattle, horses and chickens in Germany more than 100 years ago in 1902, considered that the subject should be included in the curriculum at veterinary schools.[8] Indeed, there is a substantial

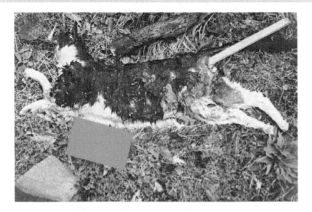

Fig. 14.1 – Post-mortem examination of this markedly decomposed cat was unable to ascertain whether the stick had been inserted into the anus before or after death. Irrespective of this uncertainty, the action of inserting the object is considered sexual in nature. (By kind permission of the Scottish Society for the Prevention of Cruelty to Animals.)

body of published reports (particularly on farmed livestock and horses) in several European languages. (For references, see Berchtold & Prechtl 2004.[9])

Farmed livestock

The injuries documented in farmed livestock tend to be those associated with insertion of a foreign body into the vagina or anus. Reichert[8] pointed out that penile penetration in large animals would not cause injury but that the insertion of an implement would do so.

In 2004 Berchtold & Prechtl[9] described the cases of three dairy cows (on the same farm) with symptoms of acute localised peritonitis, which was caused by 'punch-type' rectal injuries, and in 2006 Hvozdik and colleagues[10] described the fatal violent sexual abuse of five female calves, in which the vagina and rectum of each animal had been traumatised by a glass bottle.

In 1934 Zanni[11] pointed out that, although it can be very simple to detect a traumatic wound in the rectum, this does depend on the size of the implement used. In cases where a nail or similar object is employed, it may be difficult to detect this at post-mortem examination.

Horses

Injuries caused by the insertion of an implement into the vagina and/or rectum and vagina have been well described by Reichert[8]. One such case involved a series of 20 mares who became seriously ill at irregular intervals over a period of 3 years. Meticulous investigation failed to find the cause. However, the 20th mare was found to have a wound the size of a large nail or the tip of a fork in the colon. Further investigation showed that the animals started to become ill only when one particular person began work at the premises, and the episodes stopped when this person was removed.

Rectal tears do occur in horses, the majority being iatrogenic (physician induced) as they occur during routine veterinary rectal palpation.[12] There are several other less common causes, one being rectal palpation carried out by the owner.[13,14]

Cases where horses have been slashed about the body have been considered sexual in nature. For example, in 2002 Schedel-Stupperich[15] reported that of more than 1000 violent crimes against horses in Germany between 1993 and 2000, 25% of the injuries were associated with the genitalia.

Companion animals

Detailed data on the injuries associated with the sexual abuse of companion animals are distinctly sparse. However, a study by Munro & Thrusfield[5] investigating veterinarians' perception and experience of non-accidental injury to pets in the UK identified 6% of the 448 reported cases as sexual in nature: *'This suggests that the problem is not trivial'* (p 336).

There were 21 cases in dogs (14 females and seven males), five in cats (three females, one male, and one of unspecified sex), and two in which the species and sex were not identified but the injuries involved the vagina and perianal area respectively.

The types of injury reported included vaginal and anorectal penetrative penile injury, injury caused by insertion of a variety of implements, perianal trauma, penetrating wounds around the anus or vulva, trauma to the female genitalia (vulva, vagina, uterus) and trauma to the male genitalia, including ligatures around the penis or scrotum. Two animals (both female dogs) were reported to have no injuries.

Examination

Specialised kits (sometimes referred to as 'rape kits') are available for use in the examination of human victims of sexual assault, and can also be useful in animal cases. A thorough description of their use, with details for sourcing them in the USA, is given by Sinclair and co-workers.[16] In the UK similar kits are available.[17,18]

Schudel[19] provides a description of the identification of canine spermatozoa and its differentiation from human spermatozoa. The methods employed may be useful in the investigation of cases of alleged sexual abuse where male dogs are involved.

Summary

- Be aware that sexual abuse of animals exists and that injuries can result.
- Both farmed livestock and companion animals are used.
- Female *and* male animals may be affected.

- The injuries involve the genitalia and the anus and rectum.
- Include sexual abuse in the differential diagnosis of lesions affecting the genitalia, the anus and the rectum (in birds, in injuries affecting the cloaca).
- As with non-accidental injury (see Chapter 3), the circumstances must also be taken into consideration. For example, there may be an inconsistent history that does not fit with the injury.

References

1. Beetz A. Love, violence, and sexuality in relationships between humans and animals. Dissertation, University of Erlangen-Nürnberg. Aachen: Shaker; 2002.
2. Beirne P. Rethinking bestiality: towards a concept of interspecies assault. Theor Criminol 1997; 1:317–340.
3. Miletski H. Zoophilia – implications for therapy. J Sex Educ Ther 2001; 26:85–89.
4. Kowal L. Recognising animal abuse: what veterinarians can learn from the field of child abuse and neglect. In: Recognising and reporting animal abuse: a veterinarian's guide. Denver: American Humane Association; 1998:40–48.
5. Munro HMC, Thrusfield M. 'Battered pets': sexual abuse. J Small Anim Pract 2001; 42:333–337.
6. Duffield G, Hassiotis A, Vizard E. Zoophilia in young sexual abusers. J Forensic Psychiatry 1998; 9:294–304.
7. Hentig H. Soziologie der zoophilen Neigung. In: Burger-Prinz H, Giese H, eds. Beiträge zur Sexualforschung. Stuttgart: Enke; 1962.
8. Reichert F. Die Bedeutung der sexuellen Psychopathie des Menschen für die Tierheilkunde. Vet Med Diss, University of Berne, Munich; 1902.
9. Berchtold J, Prechtl J. Perforierende Mastdarmverletzungen bei drei Rindern– ein Fallbericht. Der Praktische Tierarzt 2004; 85:754–760.
10. Hvozdik A, Bugarský A, Kottferová J et al. Ethological, psychological, and legal aspects of animal sexual abuse. Vet J 2006; 172:374–376.
11. Zanni L. Repertorio del veterinario pratico: sulle ferite traumatiche del retto. La Clinica Veterinaria 1934; X111:835–839.
12. Freeman DE. Rectum and anus. In: Auer JA, Stick JA, eds. Equine surgery, 3rd edn. St Louis: Saunders Elsevier; 2006:479–481.
13. Welland L. Transmural rectal intestinal evisceration associated with parturition in a primiparous mare. Can Vet J 2003; 44:740–742.
14. Reece D. Rectal rupture in a mare. Aust Vet Pract 1981; 11:140–142.
15. Schedel-Stupperich A. Schwere Gewaltdelikte an Pferden – Phänomenologie, psychosoziales Konstrukt. Deutsche Tierärztliche Wochenschrift 2002; 109:116–119.
16. Sinclair L, Merck M, Lockwood R. Animal sexual assault. In: Forensic investigation of animal cruelty. A guide for veterinary and law enforcement professionals. Washington, DC: Humane Society Press; 2006:173–178.
17. The Forensic Science Service®. Online. Available: http://www.forensic.gov.uk 23 July 2007.
18. Scenesafe® evidence recovery systems. Online. Available: http://www.scenesafe.co.uk 23 July 2007.
19. Schudel D. Screening for canine spermatozoa. Sci Justice 2001; 41:117–119.

15 | Poisoning

Introduction

Excellent texts on veterinary toxicology and poisoning of domestic animals and free-living species are available.[1-6] This short chapter makes no attempt to provide a guide to poisons and their effects, but merely addresses a number of practical issues related to the investigation of alleged poisonings.

The first issue in suspect 'poisoning' cases is why poisoning is being considered. Are there aspects of the history that place poisoning high on the differential diagnosis list? – for example, 5000 dead fish downstream of a chemical plant. Or is 'poisoning' a tentative diagnosis based on inability to find an alternative cause of death in an otherwise healthy looking animal?

The source of the toxic product may, initially, be obscure, as in the case of percutaneous absorption of phenolics from pentachlorophenol-treated wood shaving used for bedding.[7] Similarly, suspicious deaths in cage birds may be related to inadvertent poisoning caused by overheating of cooking ware coated with polytetrafluoroethylene (PTFE) or by acrolein or other vapours associated with cooking fats and oils.[8]

Toxicity related to environmental contamination may be a natural phenomenon or one linked to the ingestion of discarded human-made objects such as shotgun pellets, lead fishing weights or vehicle batteries. Other poisonings result from carelessness, such as allowing dogs to have access to slug baits or cats to lap spilled ethylene glycol. On farms, spilled insecticides or over-enthusiastic application of agrochemicals pose a threat to wildlife.

Malicious poisoning of wildlife and domestic animals – raptors, foxes, dogs and cats – is depressingly common and often involves agrochemicals or rodenticides. These deliberate poisonings rely on the target species, or individual, taking bait. Examples are dead rabbits contaminated with carbofuran (Fig. 15.1), or eggs laced with strychnine or organophosphorus insecticide. These baits are, however, indiscriminate and it may be a family dog out for a walk with the children that finds and consumes the poison.

Initial preparations

Standard operative procedures (SOP) in the post-mortem room serve to avoid cross-contamination and give the authorities confidence that the best possible samples were retrieved for analysis:

- Agree a protocol with a toxicology laboratory that subscribes to a third-party quality assurance scheme.
- Determine which analyses the laboratory is able to conduct.
- Prepare sampling kits with the appropriate containers, e.g. chemically clean glass bottles, blood tubes, etc.
- Prepare a list of the conditions under which the various samples should be stored and handled before arrival at the toxicology laboratory, e.g. +4°C, −80°C.
- Confirm delivery details and 'out-of-hours' arrangements, ensuring that the chain of evidence can be maintained.
- Contact the toxicology laboratory before commencing the post-mortem examination.

Post-mortem examination

When more than one animal is involved it is essential that gloves, aprons, instruments and the covering of the post-mortem room table are changed between animals.

1. Many poisons are ingested and any material in the mouth, crop, oesophagus and stomach should be collected. The mouth and crop/oesophageal contents can be pooled, whereas the stomach contents are best collected separately.
2. As a routine, collect liver and kidney (in separate containers) plus any specific samples, e.g. blubber, as appropriate. Blood may be retrieved from the ventricles or the internal iliac veins.
3. *Change instruments and gloves between each organ sampled.*
4. Store duplicates of the samples submitted to the toxicology laboratory in the refrigerator or freezer.
5. Label, sign and date each bottle. State case number, species and organ on the container.
6. Provide a short history on the submission form and list every container being submitted, together with its contents.
7. Give as precise a steer as possible to the toxicologist regarding the type of poisoning suspected. For example, a buzzard in good bodily condition found dead with considerable quantities of food in the mouth and crop might suggest alpha-chloralose intoxication. The laboratory might then decide to run a standard set of tests focusing on chemicals

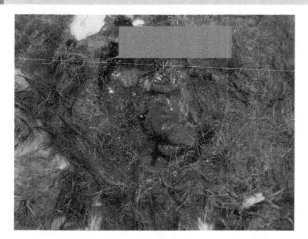

Fig. 15.1 – Note blue-coloured carbofuran granules in and around a hole in the side of a dead rabbit left on hillside as bait for raptors.

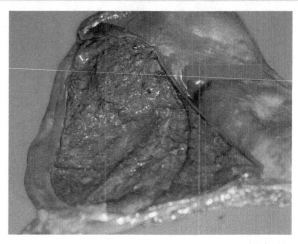

Fig. 15.2 – Stomach contents of female Belgian Shepherd dog poisoned by metaldehyde.

available to estate managers and farmers. Alternatively, when a buzzard has partially digested portions of mice or rats in the stomach, the tests might include anticoagulant rodenticides to investigate the possibility of secondary poisoning.

8. In specific cases, toxicological analysis might be delayed pending the results of other laboratory tests. In suspected ethylene glycol poisoning, for example, histopathological examination of the kidney might be considered a useful first step.

During the post-mortem examination, colour changes to the gastrointestinal contents can provide clues to the possible nature of the poison (Fig. 15.2). However, the blue colour of carbofuran granules tends to leach from the granules when they are in the stomach, causing them to assume a less obvious off-white hue.

References

1. Campbell A, Chapman M. Handbook of poisoning of dogs and cats. Oxford: Blackwell Science; 2000.

2. Murphy M. Field guide to common animal poisons. Ames: Iowa State University Press; 1996.

3. Peterson ME, Tolcott PA. Small animal toxicology. Philadelphia: W B Saunders; 2001.

4. Plumlee KH. Clinical veterinary toxicology. St Louis: Mosby; 2004.

5. Roder JD. Veterinary toxicology. Boston: Butterworth-Heinemann; 2001.

6. Fairbrother A, Locke LN, Hoff GL. Non-infectious diseases of wildlife, 2nd edn. London: Manson Publishing; 1996.

7. Foster D. Poison. Phenolics. In Practice 1994; 16:330–331.

8. Duff P. Acute inhalant toxicoses of cagebirds. Vet Rec 1997; 141:107.

Index

Note: Page numbers in *italics* refer to pictures.

Edwards Brothers Malloy
Ann Arbor MI. USA
July 20, 2016